Effective
HEALTH RISK
MESSAGES

Kim Witte__

Gary Meyer__

Dennis Martell__

Effective
HEALTH RISK
MESSAGES

A Step-by-Step Guide

Sage Publications
International Educational and Professional Publisher
Thousand Oaks ■ London ■ New Delhi

For information:

 Sage Publications, Inc.
2455 Teller Road
Thousand Oaks, California 91320
E-mail: order@sagepub.com

Sage Publications Ltd.
1 Olivers Yard, 55 City]
London EC1Y 1SP

SAGE Publications India Pvt Ltd
B-42 Panchsheel Enclave
PO Box 4109
New Dehli 110 017

Printed in the United States of America

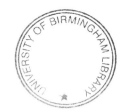

Library of Congress Cataloging-in-Publication Data

Witte, Kim.
  Effective health risk messages: A step-by-step guide /
Kim Witte, Gary Meyer, Dennis P. Martell.
      p.   cm.
  ISBN 0-7619-1508-7 (cloth: alk. paper)
  ISBN 0-7619-1509-5 (pbk.: alk. paper))
1. Health promotion. 2. Health attitudes. 3. Threat (Psychology)
4. Perception.   5. Health risk assessment. I. Meyer, Gary.
II. Martell, Dennis P. III. Title.
RA427.W67 2000
613—dc21   00-012404

02 03 04 05 10 9 8 7 6 5 4 3 2

Acquiring Editor:	Margaret H. Seawell
Production Editor:	Claudia A. Hoffman
Editorial Assistant:	Candice Crosetti
Typesetter/Designer:	Janelle LeMaster
Indexer:	Molly Hall
Cover Designer:	Michelle Lee

Contents

Preface for Instructors
and Practitioners

We designed this book for *Instructors* with the express purpose of providing students (and practitioners) with practical, theoretically based hands-on experience in designing and evaluating a health risk campaign. The book has 10 chapters to accommodate both quarter and semester systems, assuming you go through a chapter a week. It can work as a stand-alone text or as a supplemental workbook to a more traditional text. The worksheets take students step-by-step through the formative, message development, and outcome phases of a health communication campaign. Pilot tests of the worksheets indicate that students retain the material and rate classes using these worksheets as among the best they've ever taken.

For *Practitioners*, we wanted to create a resource that clearly, plainly, and concretely explained how to go about conducting a theoretically based formative and outcome evaluation, as well as how to develop theoretically based messages. The worksheets and examples used in the book can be used with your clients or target audience members. This step-by-step guide was written as a resource guidebook, as well as to provide you with ready-to-use materials for your own health communication efforts. Enjoy and Good Luck!

Acknowledgments

Thanks to Kimo Ah Yun (University of Washington), Anthony J. Roberto (Michigan State University), Dorothy Tan-Wilhelm (National Institute of Occupational Safety and Health), Susan E. Tate (University of Virginia), Mark P. Fulop (San Diego State University), Claire A. Stiles (Eckerd College), and Meagan Grant (Marquette University), for providing feedback on earlier drafts of the manuscript. Drs. Janet Lillie, Judith Berkowitz, Kenzie Cameron, Maria Lapinski, Lisa Murray-Johnson, and Wen-Ying Liu are gratefully acknowledged for their role in the research that helped form many of the ideas here. Most of all, thanks to our respective soul mates (Thom, Anne, and Colleen) for their support of this project.

1

What Are
Health Risk Messages?

We remember the first time we saw a crashed car—the kind with bloodstains on the seat and pieces of hair embedded in the broken windshield. It was parked in front of a grocery store to "remind" teenagers to avoid drinking and driving. We would peer into it, trying to imagine what those last few moments of life were like for the occupants. Did they feel the crash? How long were they alive with their heads through the windshield? What were their last moments like? We would read the vignettes about the victims' lives and what led to their deaths—usually binge drinking and then racing their cars at 80 mph down 35 mph roads. When their deaths became all too real, all too vivid, we began our morbid humor, trying to find ways to cope with the horror of it all. Later that night, we'd tell ghost stories about the dead teens and how they now haunted the junk food sections of that very grocery store.

The goal of these types of displays is to convince people to avoid drinking and driving. But why not simply tell people "don't drink and drive"? Why not just give them the facts? Are such graphic displays of the consequences of drinking and driving needed? Do we really need to scare people into doing something? Many academics and health educators say yes. They firmly believe that logical and reasoned messages fall on deaf ears. They believe you have to hook people emotionally and get them aroused before they will listen and act.

Because individuals make so many decisions based on their emotions, instead of logic, it is useful to look into the research on how emotional, persuasive messages work. Most health risk messages are "fear appeals," or persuasive messages that arouse fear to gain compliance. For example, most health risk messages try to persuade by suggesting that you'll get hurt, get a disease, or even die if you don't follow some recommended behavior. More than 45 years of research on fear appeals forms the basis for this book and provides a rich resource of information about what does and does not work in health risk messages. In this book, we explain exactly what a fear appeal is, how it's used, various theoretical perspectives, and give you the nuts-and-bolts knowledge on developing an effective health risk message.

Overall, this book is intended to move the research out of the ivory tower and into the field. As such, we have included simple and clear explanations of what works and what doesn't. We also have provided exercises and worksheets for you to develop your own campaigns or persuasive messages that fit your special needs and address the special health problems your target audiences face. Adapt what works for you and make it your own. So, let's start at the beginning—what exactly is a fear appeal?

∷ HEALTH RISK MESSAGES DEFINED

The fear appeal, commonly known as the "scare tactic," is the most common persuasive message used in health campaigns. You're probably familiar with the fear appeal and have used it many times yourself. If you've ever tried to scare people into doing what you wanted them to do, then you've used a fear appeal. Formally defined, fear appeals arouse fear by promising negative consequences for not doing a certain behavior. Because you don't want the negative consequences to occur and you are (presumably) afraid of experiencing the negative consequences, you do what's suggested in the appeal.

> **Fear Appeal**
> A persuasive message that arouses fear by outlining the negative consequences that occur if a certain action is not taken.

Fear appeals are used all of the time by lots of different groups of people. For example, doctors use fear appeals frequently with their patients when they say, "If you don't stop smoking/drinking/eating too much, then you're going to have a heart attack/high blood pressure/feel sick." Parents and teachers also use them a great deal. For example, does the following bring back any childhood memories for any of you? "If you don't clean your room, you won't be able to watch TV. If you don't finish your homework, you can't go out to recess. If you're not home by midnight, you're grounded."

Fear appeals are popular in political campaigns too. "If you don't vote for I.M. King, then unemployment will increase, the environment will disintegrate, and you'll have to pay more taxes." Fear appeals are even used in advertisements. One recent advertisement attempted to sell computers by using the fear appeal, "It's too early for children to fail. A computer prevents this." The advertisement was trying to scare parents into buying a computer by suggesting their children would fall hopelessly behind their classmates. The next time you read a popular magazine, look closely at the advertisements and you'll be surprised at just how many promise negative consequences unless their product is used.

Even though fear appeals are used in a variety of situations, they are most naturally used in health domains or domains that carry risk. People are naturally fearful of illness, disease, injuries, and death and want to stay healthy. By definition, most health risk messages are fear appeals. That is, most persuasive messages designed to promote health and prevent disease outline negative consequences that occur if a certain protective action is not taken. They attempt to arouse fear by saying you'll be hurt, get sick, or even die if you don't do what the message suggests. Thus, most health risk messages are fear appeals.

Used correctly, the fear appeal can motivate people to take care of themselves and practice healthy behaviors. However, fear appeals can and do fail if used improperly. And, sometimes even the best fear appeal (or any other kind of persuasive message, for that matter) simply doesn't work because of cultural or personality factors. Most often however, when the fear appeal doesn't work, it's because it was developed without theoretical guidance.

WHAT'S A THEORY? ■

Even though most people agree that theoretically based messages are a good idea, few actually base their messages on theories. One recent study even found that health education practitioners discount theory (Dearing et al., 1996). However, the advantages to using theoretically based campaigns are well-documented. The use of theory to develop your persuasive message saves time and money because there is less trial and error, and theoretically based campaigns are more likely to succeed compared with campaigns developed from inspiration alone (Maibach & Parrot, 1995; Rice & Atkin, 1989).

There are several reasons people don't use theories when they develop their campaigns or persuasive messages. First, some people are intimidated by theories. We have found that many don't quite know what a "theory" is. When we were starting out in this field, we too had a difficult time figuring out exactly what constituted a theory. Finally, we were told a theory was simply an explanation. More specifically, *a theory is an explanation of how different variables or factors work together to produce a certain outcome.* Thus, if a theory concerning why Joe gets good grades in college is needed, simply look for the factors or variables explaining why Joe gets good grades. The variables or factors that cause the particular outcome of Joe getting good grades in college might be (a) amount of time he studies, (b) intelligence, and (c) the quality of his high school education. Thus, the theory explaining why Joe gets good grades in college is based on a combination of the following variables:

a. Joe had an excellent high school education with college preparatory courses,

b. Joe is very intelligent with an IQ of 118, and

c. Joe spends four hours each day studying for classes.

As you can see, a theory is simply an explanation of why things occur.

Second, when people learn of a new "theory," it often seems too complex, too abstract, or too elaborate to be of any use in the "real world." Unfortunately, academics typically write for each other instead of for practitioners. The result is that many research articles are laden with difficult-to-understand jargon and advanced statistical procedures that make little sense to those outside the narrow field of persuasion. However, most academics do want to make a difference in the real world. That's why they spend much of their time developing theories. But how is a theory developed?

> **Theory**
> An explanation of how two or more variables work together to produce a certain outcome(s).

To develop a theory, researchers first isolate the variables that influence outcomes. For fear appeals, researchers first had to isolate the message features and internal psychological processes that influenced behaviors. Then, researchers must figure out how these variables should be influenced to produce certain outcomes. Should they be strengthened, minimized, emphasized, and so on? Finally, researchers must determine how these variables work together to influence behaviors. The final result is a theory. Thus, a theory identifies important variables, tells you whether they should be strong or weak (high or low), and tells you how the variables work together to influence outcomes.

Even though theories may seem complex, if you use them to guide the development of your persuasive message, you actually save time. You cut the guesswork. With a theory, you know which variables to focus on, how to emphasize these variables in the proper direction, and how these variables work together to produce a certain outcome, in this case, adoption of a recommended response. Once you become familiar with a theory, you are able to generate effective persuasive messages in a more efficient manner.

Our goal in this book is to translate how to use a fear appeal theory in your everyday work. By using a theory, you increase your chances of developing persuasive messages that work and decrease the amount of time and money needed to make your projects successful. The theory we present in Chapter 2 can be used for any persuasive message, whether it's an interpersonal message between you and a client or a mediated message broadcast over television. Before we talk about the theory however, let's talk about what makes up a fear appeal.

■■ THE COMPONENTS OF A FEAR APPEAL

The modern fear appeal typically has two components—the threat and the recommended response. The threat portion of the message usually outlines the negative consequences that occur if you don't do what's advocated. The recommended response is what you should do to avoid experiencing the threat.

Figure 1.1 is a good example of a fear appeal used in an advertisement. First, the advertisers try to scare you by outlining the terrible things that can happen in baby's clothes. Thus, the threat portion of this fear appeal is clearly outlined as, "baby's clothes can be a breeding ground for germs. Germs that cause staph infections, diaper rash, and other skin irritations. Detergents alone can't kill these germs." (Wow! Did you ever hear of a baby getting a staph infection from dirty clothes? It's a wonder we all survived infancy.)

Then, the fear appeal gives a specific recommended response, "But Clorox Liquid Bleach removes over 99% of the germs that can cause these infections and irritations. Germs detergents alone leave behind." (Whew! I was getting worried about my baby, but now I have a solution that looks safe and effective. I think I'll go buy some Clorox.) Thus, purchasing Clorox Liquid Bleach is the behavioral response the advertisers are trying to inspire by scaring you about what happens if you don't buy Clorox.

Another example of a fear appeal is shown in Figure 1.2. In this fear appeal, the threat and the recommended response are not as cleanly divided as in the Clorox fear appeal. Here, you have to read the whole message to learn that the negative consequences experienced by a "couch potato" are "wear and tear on heart" and "heart disease and stroke." You have to work a little bit harder to figure out exactly what the threat is in this fear appeal. However, if you are familiar with American culture, you probably already know that couch potatoes are known to suffer heart disease, cancer, and generally poor health. The recommended response in this fear appeal is clearly stated, *"Now is the time to teach your kids good habits. Like eating low-fat, low-cholesterol foods. And getting plenty of exercise."* There's even a toll-free number to call to get more information.

These two examples of fear appeals show that typically these messages contain a threat component and a recommended response component. Sometimes the threat and recommended response sections are clearly identifiable, as in Figure 1.1. Sometimes the threat and recommended response sections are mixed together, as in Figure 1.2. In addition, some fear appeals offer multiple responses. While Figure 1.1 simply urges you to buy Clorox Liquid Bleach to solve your problem, Figure 1.2 gives diet and exercise advice and even includes a 1-800 number to call to get more specific information on how

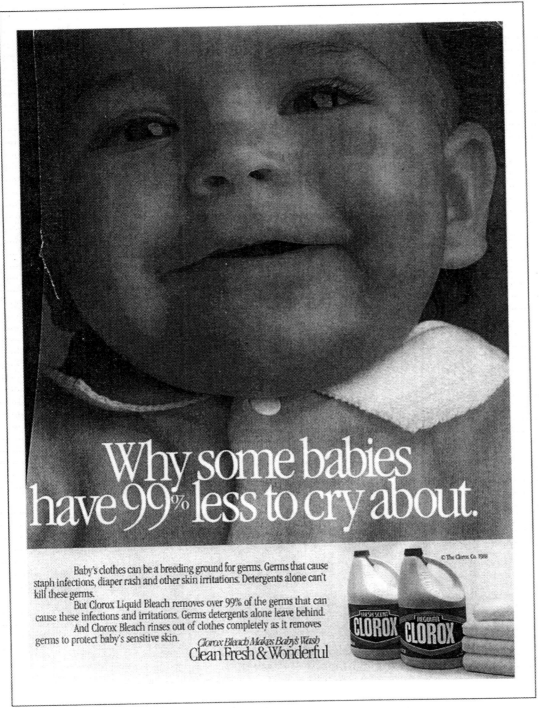

Why some babies have 99% less to cry about.

Baby's clothes can be a breeding ground for germs. Germs that cause staph infections, diaper rash and other skin irritations. Detergents alone can't kill these germs.

But Clorox Liquid Bleach removes over 99% of the germs that can cause these infections and irritations. Germs detergents alone leave behind.

And Clorox Bleach rinses out of clothes completely as it removes germs to protect baby's sensitive skin.

Clorox Bleach Makes Baby's Wash
Clean Fresh & Wonderful

Figure 1.1   Clorox Liquid Bleach advertisement
SOURCE: Reproduced with permission of the Clorox Company.

to carry out the recommended responses. Fear appeals aren't just limited to print advertisements. Watch television or listen to your doctor, and you'll probably hear and see fear appeals through them, too.

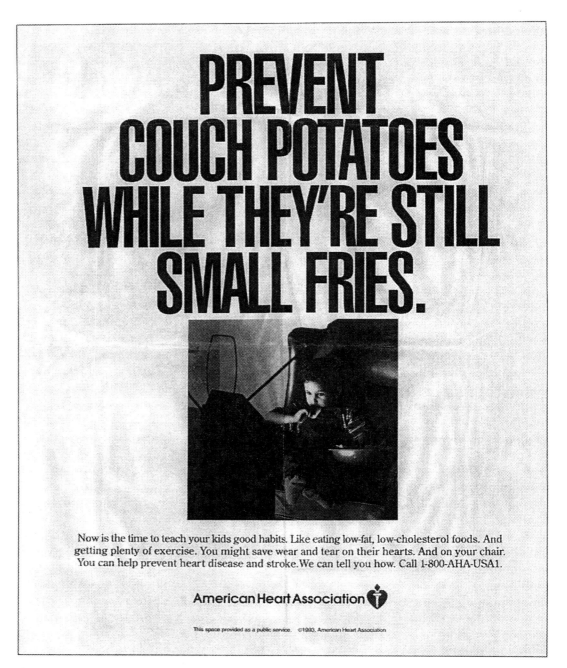

Figure 1.2 American Heart Association public service announcement
SOURCE: Reproduced with permission. Copyright © 1993, American Heart Association.

■■ EXPLICIT VERSUS IMPLICIT MESSAGES

Figure 1.3 shows probably the most widely known fear appeal, the frying egg as a description of "your brain on drugs." But here, the threat is not as clearly stated as in the Clorox advertisement. You have to figure out from the text and pictures exactly what the threat is. After studying the picture, you probably come to the conclusion that the threat is "my brains will fry if I use drugs." However, where's the recommended response? It's not explicitly stated. It is assumed that you'll draw the appropriate conclusion yourself, which is something similar to "don't use drugs" or "stop using drugs."

The recommended response portion of this fear appeal is known as an *implicit* message. Implicit messages are thought to be understood from the context of the message, although they are not clearly expressed. An *explicit* message, in contrast, is so clearly stated, there is no doubt as to its meaning. The threat portion of the message in Figure 1.3 appears more implicit than explicit. For example, if one is not familiar with the cultural colloquialism of "frying one's brains" as having a negative connotation, then one may have a difficult time understanding the point of the message.

Explicit threat messages clearly lay out the negative consequences that occur if the recommended response is not followed. Messages such as "AIDS Kills" or "More people have died from car accidents with drunk drivers than all the Americans killed in World War I, World War II, the Korean War, and the Vietnam War combined—drinking and driving is deadly" are all examples of explicitly stated threats. Messages with implicit threats are usually more subtle and simply imply a threat, but do not clearly state the negative consequences; Figure 1.3 is an example of an implicit message.

Similarly, explicit recommended response messages give specific recommendations about what to do to avoid the threat. For example, "wear a bicycle helmet," "eat bran," or "vote for Smith" are all explicit recommended response messages. In contrast, implicit messages don't give a recommended response. They assume you know what the recommended response is and will act on it. Often, smoking prevention messages have implicit recommended responses where the persuasive message outlines the dangers of cigarette smoking and simply leaves it at that. The messages don't tell you what to do and assume that if you know the dangers of cigarette smoking, you'll instinctively know that the recommended response is, "quit smoking" or "don't start smoking."

We have found that explicit recommended responses work far better than implicit recommended responses. Even though it may seem obvious that a persuasive message outlining the dangers of smoking would motivate one to not start cigarette smoking (or to quit if one already smokes), we have found that people often don't draw that conclusion. It's best to explicitly state what you want them to do. For example, we have found that a message emphasizing the terrible things that can happen to you from drinking and driving simply convinces you that drinking and driving leads to terrible things. Or, it simply convinces you that drinking and driving is bad, but it doesn't convince *you* to do something to prevent yourself from experiencing these negative consequences. Therefore, it is critical to be clear about what you want people to do to avoid experiencing the negative consequences. And, be sure to state your recommended response in a clear, easy-to-understand and easy-to-do manner.

THE USE OF CULTURALLY BASED COLLOQUIALISMS ■■

The fear appeals in Figures 1.2 and 1.3 indicate that their authors relied heavily on American cultural colloquialisms. A colloquialism is an informal phrase used to describe something within a certain cultural group. For example, every group has its own lingo, its own jargon, that is immediately understandable to the members of that group, but may be incomprehensible to people outside that group. The use of terms such as "couch potato" in Figure 1.2 and the message of "frying one's brain" in Figure 1.3 may be meaningless to members of other cultures. Thus, it is important in writing a fear appeal to make

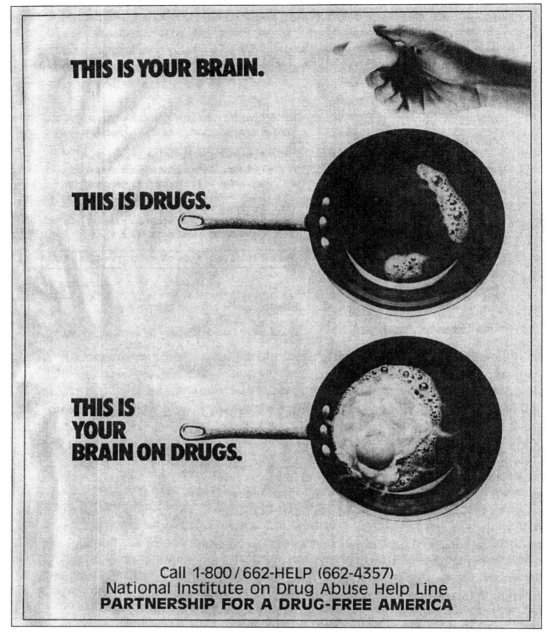

Figure 1.3 Partnership for a Drug-Free America public service announcement
SOURCE: Reproduced with permission of Partnership for a Drug-Free America.

sure the colloquialisms or lingo used to express threats or recommended responses are clearly understood by members of your target audience, that is, the audience you are trying to reach. For most Americans, these phrases are easily understood and add some humor to the fear appeal. However, if these fear appeals were shown to people living in China or Russia, they might not be understood. If you're going to use any colloquial language in your persuasive message, we recommend testing it in advance to ensure your audience clearly understands what you mean.

TYPES OF THREATS ▪▪

A fear appeal can focus on many different kinds of threats. Each of the fear appeal examples discussed so far focuses on physical harm or the physical consequences of not complying with the message. However, social threats, psychological threats, economic threats, threats to values or ethics, spiritual threats, and so on, are used to arouse fear to gain compliance. Some people fear physical harm more than anything. For these people, the typical fear appeal promising death or poor health as a result of not behaving in a certain way would probably work best. However, for other people, economic threats arouse more fear. For still others, social threats greatly outweigh any other kind. This is especially true for teenagers.

We once did a study with inner-city teen mothers. We were trying to determine the best kind of persuasive message to prevent teen pregnancy. Most of the messages we showed the teens focused on the negative consequences of early sexual intercourse. "If you have sex, you'll get pregnant. Use a condom to prevent pregnancy." The messages all assumed that "getting pregnant" was a terrible threat to the teens; pregnancy would be seen as something negative. To our surprise, however, pregnancy was often seen as a benefit of sexual intercourse. These teen girls romanticized pregnancy and motherhood and fantasized about having a baby that would love them unconditionally. To these teens, getting pregnant was not a threat!

When asked about the negative consequences of getting pregnant, the teens offered a virtually unanimous response—"losing one's friends" and "getting fat." These socially related threats were seen as devastating, and the teens uniformly had great fears about them. Thus, these findings suggested that an effective fear appeal to prevent teen pregnancy should focus on how much weight one gains when pregnant and how one might lose friends after having a baby while in high school. These social threats appear to arouse more fear and motivate recommended behaviors more than physical threats for teens.

Figure 1.4 shows a fear appeal that focuses on yet another kind of threat—a threat to one's values or ethics. This advertisement appeared in the *Utne Reader*, a magazine known to appeal to environmentalists and social liberals. Social liberals tend to boycott the tobacco industry because they believe it promotes a product that is a known health hazard to young people and children. This advertisement was appealing to that liberal audience, trying to scare readers into thinking that they might be inadvertently supporting the tobacco industry through their investments. Thus, the threat was to one's values or ethical beliefs (i.e., "supporting an entity you believe is harmful"—the tobacco industry), and the recommended response was to call for your free guide to what your investments were supporting.

Overall, one can see there are many different kinds of threats that a fear appeal can emphasize. Chapter 5's worksheets help determine the kind of threat most appropriate for a specific fear appeal. But for now, it's just important to remember that fear appeals can effectively utilize a variety of threats.

SUMMARY ▪▪

Why do so many advertisers, politicians, and parents use fear appeals? Because they work. However, as we pointed out earlier, fear appeals can and do fail if not used properly. In the next chapter, you learn about what makes fear appeals work and what makes them

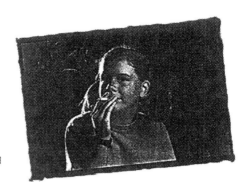

Does your retirement money go places you never dreamed of?

Great for IRAs

If you're like most people, you aren't sure what kind of investments your company or organization's retirement program is making with your money. So you might be supporting companies and industries you'd never want to.

Like tobacco. In a recent survey conducted by Co-op America, nine of the largest 15 mutual funds listed tobacco companies as one of their top ten holdings.

So make sure you know what you own. In 1982, Calvert Group began offering mutual funds that invest in socially and environmentally responsible companies. Now we've created the "Know What You Own" investor service to help you find out what companies you own through your mutual funds. Visit our service on the internet at http://www.calvertgroup.com.

And to find out how you can get your employer to offer a tobacco-free option in your retirement plan, call your financial professional or Calvert Group and ask for our free guide *Kicking the Habit.*

For your free guide, call 800-987-4873.

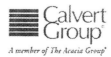

A member of The Acacia Group

KNOW WHAT YOU OWN

Calvert Distributors, Inc., 4550 Montgomery Avenue, Bethesda, MD 20814

READER SERVICE 510

Figure 1.4 Calvert Group investment advertisement
SOURCE: Reproduced with permission, Calvert Distributors, Inc.

fail. In this chapter, we defined what a fear appeal is, outlined its components, and talked about the advantages of using theoretically based messages. In addition, we discussed the value of explicit versus implicit messages, the use of colloquialisms in fear appeals, and the types of threats used to arouse fear. In the worksheets section for Chapter 1, there are three worksheets that test your understanding of these concepts.

2

History of
Health Risk Messages

Fear Appeal Theories from 1953 to 1991

The formal study of health risk messages began in the early 1950s when researchers at Yale University examined the influence of fear-arousing dental hygiene messages on high school students' tooth-brushing behavior (Janis & Feshbach, 1953). The messages used in this study described health risks ranging from mild physical threats such as toothaches, sore and inflamed gums, and cavities, to extremely severe physical threats such as cancer, blindness, and paralysis (all from not brushing your teeth properly). The Yale University researchers were interested in studying a wide variety of message appeals; fear appeals were just one of many message types they studied. In the case of fear appeals, it was recognized that the easiest way to arouse fear was to threaten physical harm. Thus, as is the case now, nearly all of the early fear appeal research naturally focused on topics where threats easily could be made to one's health.

Many of the early fear appeal scholars at Yale University were also involved in developing the Health Belief Model, a popular concept describing health behaviors (see Rosenstock, 1974). Given the similarities between the variables in fear appeal theories and those in the Health Belief Model, some researchers have gone so far as to suggest that fear appeal research is simply an experimental variant of the Health Belief Model (Prentice-Dunn & Rogers, 1986; more on the Health Belief Model in Chapter 4). Those familiar with the Health Belief Model will notice similarities between it and fear appeal theories.

In this chapter, we start at the beginning and examine fear appeal theories from their first formalization. Specifically, we focus on the three dominant approaches to fear appeals from 1953 to the 1990s (Dillard, 1994; Witte, 1992a). These theories represent the major research on health risk messages during this time period. Then, in Chapter 3, we present the Extended Parallel Process Model (EPPM), which integrates these earlier perspectives and represents current theorizing on how people process health risk messages.

■■ FEAR-AS-ACQUIRED DRIVE MODEL

Health risk messages in the form of fear-arousing messages first began to be studied in the early 1950s by a group of scholars at Yale University (Hovland, Janis, & Kelly, 1953; Janis, 1967). The dominant theories of this time were "learning theories," which often used a system of rewards to reinforce certain behaviors. These scholars adopted that perspective and proposed that first people need to learn about a certain risk or threat, and then they need to be taught to fear it. They said that people learned to fear a threat through persuasive messages.

These scholars believed that fear was a powerful drive that would motivate action. They reasoned that fear was a negative drive, an unpleasant state, and that people would want to get rid of that unpleasant feeling of fear. They then proposed offering specific behaviors in the message that, if performed, would eliminate the threat and presumably the fear. If fear were eliminated by the performance of a specific behavior, then the performance of that behavior would be seen as "rewarding" because it removed the unpleasant state of fear. Because the performance of that behavior was rewarding (it eliminated fear), it would become the "learned" and habitual response to the health threat. That is, any time people were faced with that health threat, they would perform the recommended behavior because it was rewarding to do so. An example may prove useful here.

Imagine a severe flu outbreak in your city. The public health officials want everyone to get vaccinated so they are protected against this particular strain. The severe flu is the threat and getting vaccinated is the recommended response. Using the fear-as-acquired drive model, health educators would first educate the public about this particular strain of flu and its terrible impact on one's health (vomiting, diarrhea, fatigue). They would try to arouse fear about the flu by offering stories of the effects on those infected, such as dropping out of school or even death. You realize you are at risk for getting this strain of the flu and this scares you. You want to stay healthy so you can go to Florida over spring break. Now you're motivated to act. Your fear has motivated you to do something.

You realize that you saw a billboard with a toll-free number about where to get vaccinations for only $5. You call and receive your shot and feel so relieved, your fear is gone. Every winter from this point on, whenever the threat of flu is raised, you simply go get a vaccination. Getting a vaccination (the recommended response) has become your reinforced, habitual response to the threat of flu. According to the fear-as-acquired drive model, it became your habitual response because the vaccination removed your fear; because it got rid of your fear, the vaccination against the flu was rewarding and reinforcing.

Now, what happens if the recommended response *does not* eliminate the fear? According to the fear-as-acquired drive model, other responses would be tried, such as maladaptive psychological strategies including denial of the threat, defensive avoidance, reactance, and so on, until one of these reduced the fear. Whatever response reduced the fear would become the reinforced, habitual response to the threat. Thus, if you were fearful about getting the flu and couldn't get to a clinic for a shot, you would still be motivated to get rid of your fear. You might try some psychological responses, such as:

- Denial of threat: "I don't believe there's really an epidemic, I don't know anyone with the flu."
- Defensive avoidance: "I'm just not going to think about it, there's no use worrying about it."
- Reactance: "This is just another silly government announcement; they're just trying to get more money from us."

If one of these responses eliminated your fear, then it would become your habitual, reinforced response to the threat of flu. Thus, if you were faced with another flu epidemic where the recommended response was vaccination, you would ignore that recommendation and simply deny that there was really a problem, because this is now your habitual response to any flu epidemic message.

In summary, according to the Fear-as-Acquired Drive Model, the trick is to arouse enough fear to motivate action, but just enough so the recommended response eliminates the fear and becomes the reinforced response (Janis, 1967). If the recommended response does not eliminate the fear, then health educators risk having other responses becoming reinforced responses to the health threat—a dangerous situation because once a response works in reducing fear, it becomes habitual and consequentially, is more difficult to change.

Overall, the Fear-as-Acquired Drive Model proposed a curvilinear relationship between fear and behavior change, such that a moderate amount of fear led to the greatest behavior change. Figure 2.1 shows that initially, as fear arousal increases, so does the probability of acceptance of a message's recommendations. For each topic and/or person, there is an optimal amount of fear arousal. Too little fear does not provide enough motivation to adopt the recommended response, and too much fear causes rejection of the message (see different optimal levels in Figure 2.1). When fear arousal exceeds the optimal level, the fear-as-acquired drive suggests that respondents cannot adequately eliminate their fear through performance of the recommended response. As a result, maladaptive responses are used to reduce the fear. Overall, Figure 2.1 illustrates Janis's (1967) premise that a moderate amount of fear led to the greatest amount of message acceptance.

The Fear-as-Acquired Drive Model decreased in popularity in the late 1960s because further studies showed that as fear increased, so did attitude or behavior change (Dabbs & Leventhal, 1966; Higbee, 1969; Leventhal, Jones, & Trembly, 1966; Leventhal & Niles, 1964; Leventhal & Trembly, 1968; Leventhal, Singer, & Jones, 1965; Leventhal & Watts, 1966; Leventhal, Watts, & Pagano, 1967). These studies contradicted Janis's (1967) hypothesis that a moderate amount of fear worked best and too much fear caused messages to be rejected. Further, these and other studies showed that the reduction of fear—an essential component of the Fear-as-Acquired-Drive Model—was not necessary for behavior change (Giesen & Hendrick, 1974; Hendrick, Giesen, & Borden, 1975; Mewborn & Rogers, 1979; Rogers, 1983; Rogers & Deckner, 1975). You could have high levels of fear *and* high levels of attitude and behavior change. Howard Leventhal, a professor at Yale University at the time, provided the next leap in theories on how fear appeals work.

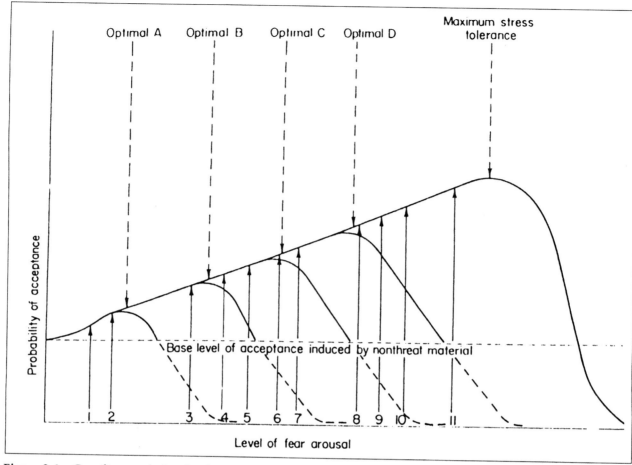

Figure 2.1 Curvilinear relationship between fear and behavior change
SOURCE: Janis, 1967. Reprinted with permission of Academic Press.

■■ THE PARALLEL PROCESS MODEL

Leventhal (1970, 1971) proposed that two distinct processes occurred in response to health risk messages. He argued that previous research had focused on emotional processes such as fear arousal and fear reduction. But, he said, cognitive processes also occurred, in which people thought about the threat or danger and strategies to avert the threat. He called the former the "fear control process" and the latter, the "danger control process." Leventhal said that when people engaged in danger control processes, or *thought* about the danger and ways to control it, then they were likely to make recommended behavioral changes and protect themselves against the danger. That is, they would "control the danger." In contrast, when people engaged in fear control processes, or focused on controlling their *feelings*, then they would be more likely to engage in maladaptive processes to "control their fear" and ignore the danger.

Think of a situation in which you were faced with a grave threat. Sometimes, you may have tried to control the danger by thinking about your risk of experiencing the threat and ways to avoid it. If you did this, you engaged in the danger control process. Now, think of times when your fear was so overwhelming that you didn't even think of the threat. Instead, you focused on ways to calm down your racing heart, your sweaty palms, and your nervousness. You may have taken some deep breaths, drunk some water, or smoked a cigarette. These all are fear control strategies. You were controlling your fear, but without any thought of the actual danger facing you.

Leventhal's (1970, 1971) ideas moved fear appeal research forward significantly by separating the cognitive from the emotional responses. However, although he suggested general states describing fear and danger control processes, he did not specify when one would dominate over the other. While researchers have criticized the Parallel Process Model's lack of precision (e.g., Beck & Frankel, 1981), it is clear that it offers a useful way of viewing responses to health risk messages.

PROTECTION MOTIVATION THEORY ■■

Ronald Rogers focused in on the "danger control" side of Leventhal's Parallel Process Model. Specifically, he explored people's cognitive, or thought-based, reactions to health risk messages. His model, called the Protection Motivation Theory (PMT), was the first to identify the components of a health risk message. Rogers suggested that most health risk messages talked about

a. the probability that a threat would occur,
b. the magnitude of noxiousness if the threat occurred, and
c. the effectiveness of the recommended response to avert the threat.

He stated that these message components led to "corresponding cognitive mediators," or corresponding perceptions, related to each component.

As shown in Figure 2.2, PMT suggests that message descriptions about the probability of a threat occurring lead to perceptions of one's vulnerability or susceptibility to the threat. For example, how much does the message make you feel at risk for actually experiencing the threat? Second, message statements about the magnitude of noxiousness of a threat lead to perceptions about the severity of the threat. For example, does the message make you think the threat is serious and significant or small and trivial? Finally, message descriptions of the recommended response lead to perceptions of the "response efficacy" of the recommendation. For example, does the message make you believe the recommended response would work, that is, effectively avert the threat?

Rogers (1975) hypothesized that when the components of the fear appeal message caused high levels of the corresponding cognitive mediators (i.e., perceptions of severity, expectancy of exposure, and belief in the efficacy of the coping response), then "protection motivation" would be elicited, causing self-protective behavior changes. That is, if the message made one feel vulnerable to a serious and significant threat and made one believe the recommended response protected against the threat, then one would be motivated to make the necessary behavioral changes. For example, if a message made you feel that you were very likely to contract lung cancer if you smoked (vulnerability), that lung cancer was a serious health threat leading to death (severity), and that quitting smoking would prevent lung cancer (response efficacy), then according to PMT, you would be motivated to protect yourself and quit smoking. Rogers (1975) noted that protection motivation "is an intervening variable that has the typical characteristics of a motive: it arouses, sustains, and directs activity" (p. 98). Simply, PMT states the in-

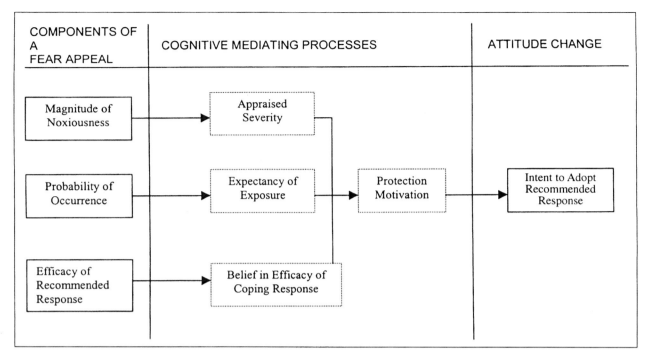

Figure 2.2 Protection Motivation Theory

SOURCE: *Journal of Psychology*, Vol. 91, p. 99, 1975. Reprinted with permission of the Helen Dwight Reid Educational Foundation. Published by Heldref Publications, 1319 Eighteenth St., NW, Washington, DC 20036-1802. Copyright © 1975.

tention of a person to perform a recommended response is a function of how much protection motivation is elicited by the cognitive mediating processes of vulnerability, severity, and response efficacy.

In 1983, Rogers revised PMT (Figure 2.3). In our opinion, the revised model is not as useful to health educators as the original because of its complexity (see critique in Witte, 1992, 1998). The revised version of PMT identifies maladaptive threat appraisal and adaptive coping appraisal processes. The threat appraisal process is called maladaptive because it leads to decreases in motivation to protect oneself. The coping appraisal process is called adaptive because it leads to increases in the motivation to protect oneself. The revised PMT also added a new variable, self-efficacy (beliefs about one's ability to do the recommended response), which was thought to work with response efficacy to influence outcomes.

In the maladaptive threat appraisal, Rogers argues that perceptions of severity and vulnerability are subtracted from any rewards that come from performing an unhealthy behavior in the threat appraisal process. So, if rewards exceed vulnerability and severity perceptions, then maladaptive responses to the threat occur, and self-protective behavior does not. In other words, if you feel vulnerable to lung cancer and consider lung cancer to be a serious threat (high severity + high vulnerability), but you feel the rewards of smoking—such as reducing anxiety, fitting in with your peers, maintaining a low weight, and so on—are stronger than the threat, then you'll continue to smoke and place yourself at risk for lung cancer, what Rogers and others consider a maladaptive response.

Alternatively, in the coping appraisal process, Rogers (1983) says that perceptions of the costs of performing a recommended behavior are subtracted from perceptions of response and self-efficacy. Thus, when people hold strong response efficacy and self-

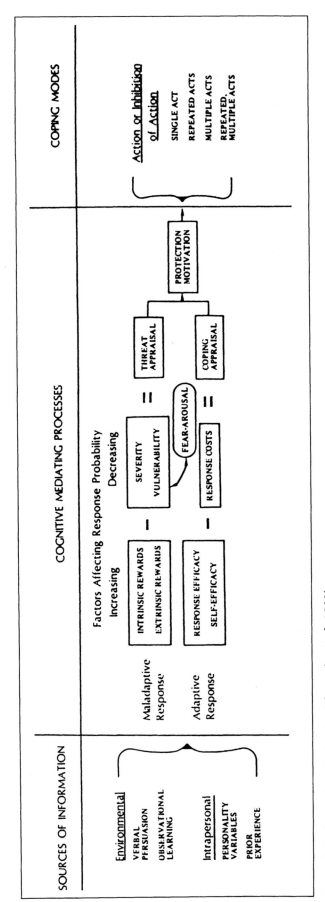

Figure 2.3 Protection Motivation Theory (revised, 1983)

SOURCE: Reprinted with permission of the Guilford Press and the author, Ronald Rogers.

efficacy beliefs and perceive that the costs of performing a recommended action are low, they engage in adaptive, self-protective responses to a health threat. In other words, if your efficacy beliefs are stronger than the costs of performing the behavior, then you'll engage in the recommended behavior. For example, if you believe quitting cigarette smoking prevents lung cancer (response efficacy), believe you can quit smoking (self-efficacy), *and* believe the costs of quitting, such as weight gain, withdrawal symptoms, cravings, and so on, are low, then you'll quit smoking cigarettes.

The relationship between the threat appraisal and the coping appraisal is said to be multiplicative, meaning that these two processes interact. In scientific terms, an interaction means that different outcomes are expected under different conditions. For example, temperature and rain interact to produce corn. As the amount of rain increases when the weather is warm, corn grows faster. However, as the amount of rain increases when the weather is cold, seedlings remain soggy and may even mildew and die. Given the same amount of rain, you get two fundamentally different outcomes depending on the weather conditions. Interactions or multiplicative relationships work the same way in the social sciences. We expect different things to happen under different conditions.

The interaction proposed in PMT is that as threat appraisal increases (i.e., perceptions of severity and vulnerability outweigh rewards) under high coping appraisal conditions (i.e., perceptions of response and self-efficacy outweigh costs), individuals engage in greater levels of adaptive behavior. Conversely, as threat appraisal increases under low coping appraisal conditions (i.e., costs outweigh perceptions of response and self-efficacy), individuals engage in greater levels of maladaptive behaviors.[1]

Mathematically, this is how the revised PMT looks:

$$[\text{Rewards} - (\text{Severity} + \text{Susceptibility})] \times [(\text{Response Efficacy} + \text{Self-Efficacy}) - \text{Costs}] = \text{Outcome}$$

The first part of the equation is the threat appraisal, and the second part is the coping appraisal. Again, these appraisals are multiplied to produce outcomes.

While we think the revised PMT is less practical to health educators than the original because of its complexity, we do think the addition of self-efficacy to the model is extremely useful. Beck and Frankel (1981) were among the first to suggest that health risk messages could be improved by addressing personal efficacy (what we call self-efficacy) in addition to response efficacy. They defined personal efficacy as "the person's expectation of being able to perform the recommended threat-coping action(s) successfully" (p. 204). Beck and Frankel went so far as to suggest that personal efficacy (i.e., self-efficacy) is more important than response efficacy in promoting healthy behaviors. We tend to agree—health educators can scare, threaten, punish, beg, lie, or bribe, but if people do not believe they can do certain behaviors (i.e., have high self-efficacy), they simply won't do them.

One additional important feature about PMT is its emphasis "upon cognitive processes and protection motivation, rather than fear as an emotion" (Rogers, 1975, p. 100). Thus, thoughts about the threat are what lead to behavior change according to PMT; fear plays a very insignificant role. Rogers (1975) suggests that adherence to recommended responses "is not mediated by or a result of an emotional state of fear, but rather is a function of the amount of protective motivation aroused by cognitive appraisal processes" (p. 100). Fear does not appear as a variable in the original PMT and appears in the revised PMT (1983) as related only to perceived severity. In the revised PMT, perceived severity and fear are reciprocally related such that one's thoughts about the severity of a threat cause fear, and one's fear about a threat heightens one's thoughts about the severity of the threat.

Overall, PMT does an excellent job identifying the components of a fear appeal model and explaining the cognitive danger control side of Leventhal's model (1970, 1971). Original PMT plus the new variable self-efficacy do a good job predicting the conditions under which fear appeals work. Specifically, when perceptions of severity, susceptibility, response efficacy, and self-efficacy are high, then people appear to accept message recommendations and make attitude, intention, and behavior changes. However, both versions of PMT fail to account for when and why people reject message recommendations.

SUMMARY ■■

Each of these theories explains some aspect of reactions to fear appeals (for critiques of each model, see Witte, 1992a, 1998). Leventhal's work (1970) offers insights into the mechanisms underlying reactions to fear appeals. Janis's (1967) theorizing provides explanations of why fear appeals sometimes fail. Rogers's (1975, 1983) research demonstrates the conditions under which fear appeals worked. However, each theory by itself does not explain in an integrated, thorough manner, the conditions under which fear appeals work and under which they fail. The Extended Parallel Process Model, presented in Chapter 3, attempts to do this.

DEFINITIONS ■■

At this point, it is critical that you thoroughly understand the language of health risk messages. In this chapter, we introduced many common health risk message concepts. Four of these concepts are particularly useful in your quest to be the world's best health educator, marketer, advertiser, or other similar professional. These concepts are severity of threat, susceptibility to threat, response efficacy, and self-efficacy. These concepts can be placed into two main categories—threat and efficacy. Table 2.1 briefly defines each concept and the term fear. Each of these concepts was also defined in the section on PMT, as well.

Threat

First, we must distinguish between actual and perceived threats. An actual threat is an objective danger that exists whether we know it or not. Perceived threat, on the other hand, implies a threat that exists only because we perceive or think that it does. This perceived threat may be real or it may be imagined. For example, as a child, one of the authors used to swim in the ocean off the coast of Southern California, going very far out (sometimes beyond the pier) before turning around and swimming back to shore. The author did not perceive any threat to her safety by swimming way beyond the shoreline. Then the movie *Jaws* came out. From that moment on, when she swam more than 50 feet from the shore, she began to imagine big monsters with large teeth swimming underneath her, and she could clearly hear the "da-da-da-da-da" soundtrack of Jaws indicating imminent attack. Actually, this threat to her safety was only perceived and not real.

Table 2.1   Definitions of Key Health Risk Message Concepts

Threat	A threat is a danger or harm that exists in the environment whether we know it or not. Perceived threat is cognitions or thoughts about that danger or harm. Perceived threat is comprised of two underlying dimensions, severity and susceptibility.
Perceived Susceptibility	Beliefs about one's risk of experiencing the threat (e.g., "I'm at risk for skin cancer because I don't use sunscreen").
Perceived Severity	Beliefs about the significance or magnitude of the threat (e.g., "Skin cancer leads to death").
Efficacy	Efficacy pertains to the effectiveness, feasibility, and ease of a recommended response in impeding or averting a threat. Perceived efficacy concerns thoughts or cognitions about its underlying dimensions, that is, response efficacy and self-efficacy.
Response Efficacy	Beliefs about the effectiveness of the recommended response in deterring the threat (e.g., "Using sunscreen consistently prevents skin cancer").
Self-Efficacy	Beliefs about one's ability to perform the recommended response to avert the threat (e.g., "I am able to use sunscreen consistently to prevent skin cancer").
Fear	Fear is an internal emotional reaction comprised of psychological and physiological dimensions that may be aroused when a serious and personally relevant threat is perceived.

In most cases however, the opposite is true. Threats to health tend to exist without people being aware of them. Prior to the 1980s, children never even considered wearing bike helmets because they did not perceive the threat of head injuries although it was surely real. Health risk messages typically focus on making people think about (i.e., perceive) actual threats to their health. Our job is to induce certain *perceptions*, because perceptions (or thoughts) are the basis of action (i.e., we have to think, "I'm going to wear a bike helmet," before we actually do so).

As Table 2.1 shows, threat is composed of two dimensions—severity and susceptibility. Susceptibility to threat refers to one's vulnerability to a threat. For example, one may be susceptible to breast cancer or heart disease because of a strong family history of these diseases. In other words, perceived susceptibility is the degree to which one feels at risk for actually experiencing the threat. More often than not, health educators and advertisers are faced with audiences who think they are invulnerable, indestructible, and invincible. (We think we are, don't you?) Much research on a psychological phenomenon known as "optimistic bias" shows that individuals underestimate the degree to which bad things can happen to them and overestimate the degree to which good things can happen to them, as compared to the amount of good and bad things that can happen to other people (Weinstein, 1980,1982). They tend to think that other people have a greater likelihood of being in car accidents or robberies, for example, than they themselves.

Severity of threat refers to the degree of harm that could possibly be experienced if a threat materialized. Severe threats are seen as more imminent (experienced sooner rather than later), more fatal, more painful, and more disfiguring. For example, dying from a heart attack is often seen as less severe than dying from AIDS because the latter is more painful, disfiguring, and imminent than the former. Motivating people to perceive a threat as severe can be just as difficult as making them realize they are susceptible to a threat. Thousands of fair-skinned teens "fake bake" each spring in tanning beds. They know they're susceptible to skin cancer but shrug it off saying, "The doctor will just freeze it off; it's no big deal." These teens do not perceive skin cancer as being a severe threat. To them, it's just a matter of removing moles.

Efficacy

Efficacy is a term that might be confusing, but it's simply a synonym for effectiveness. Thus, response efficacy refers to response effectiveness and self-efficacy refers to self-effectiveness. Efficacy always pertains to the recommended behavior or the recommended response portion of the message. Thus, we discuss either the response efficacy of the recommended behavior or one's self-efficacy toward the recommended behavior. If individuals perceive a recommended response to be effective in averting, stopping, diminishing, or avoiding a threat, then they are said to have high-response efficacy. Similarly, if individuals perceive they can perform a recommended response, then they are said to have high self-efficacy.

A variable related to self-efficacy is barriers. Barriers are typically considered to be things interfering with our performance of a certain action. Barriers may be psychological, (e.g., embarrassment), structural (e.g., lack of roads to clinics), interpersonal (e.g., partners refusing to use condoms), and so on. Common barriers to performing health actions include a lack of skills, self-confidence, knowledge, and access to the right treatment, equipment, and so on. Some disagreement exists as to whether barriers merely represent the flip side of self-efficacy and are part of the overall concept of self-efficacy, or whether they are a completely separate variable, as the Health Belief Model suggests. Because we broadly define self-efficacy as one's perceived ability to perform a given action, we see anything affecting that ability as part of the overall concept of self-efficacy. Thus, because barriers potentially influence one's perceived ability to perform an action, we see barriers to self-efficacy as an integral part of the overall concept of self-efficacy. This means that, by definition, if people have high perceived self-efficacy, they have low perceived barriers, and vice versa (if people have high perceived barriers, then they have low perceived self-efficacy). In general, inducing high levels of self-efficacy is one key to a successful intervention.

Summary

Now you are equipped with four key concepts in health risk messages. Many other concepts are also useful in developing effective health risk messages, many of which are discussed in Chapter 4. But with these four concepts as your foundation, you're on your way to developing theoretically based health risk messages that work.

NOTE ▪▪

1. Parts of revised PMT become problematic when the proposed interaction effects are examined as a whole. For example, Rogers is not clear regarding what outcomes are expected under high coping appraisal conditions (i.e., perceptions of response and self-efficacy outweigh costs) as threat appraisal decreases (i.e., rewards outweigh perceptions of severity and vulnerability). See Witte 1992 and 1998 for a full critique.

3

Putting It All Together

The Extended Parallel Process Model

When in graduate school, one of the authors gathered every article available on health risk messages and fear appeals. The collection amounted to about 100 published articles. Since then, the literature has grown rapidly and there are at least twice that many. Article after article has shown that for the most part, fear appeals are extremely effective persuasive messages. The articles of the last 20 years are especially convincing. Study after study showed that fear appeals worked with many different health topics (e.g., smoking, drinking, exercise, etc.) and with many different population groups.

Armed with this academic knowledge, the author then went to the field to work with health educators to develop public health campaigns for children in southern California. To her surprise, the health educators rejected fear appeals outright and emphatically said they didn't work. The educators refused to use them. The same experience occurred with health educators all over the country. Yet, at the same time, the most common persuasive message developed by advertising companies for public health campaigns was the fear appeal. Go figure!

So, we set out to examine this paradox and find out why practitioners thought fear appeals didn't work although at the same time, the laboratory research of the previous decades showed they did. We thought about recent empirical work on fear appeals. We pondered the previous theories. We listened to what health educators said about what worked and didn't. And then, we put all these different perspectives together and came up with an explanation for when and why health risk messages work and when and why they don't.

We noticed that previous fear appeal theories had simply focused on what worked, what led people to change their health-related behavior. But these earlier theories and studies ignored what didn't work. For example, in many studies, only some people changed their behaviors in response to the message, and the study's results and discussions focused on these people. However, the articles ignored the large number of study participants who didn't change their behavior. However, to be useful, a theory needs to explain failures as well as successes. We can learn a great deal from our failures—such as what not to do in the future! So, we developed a theory that explains both successes and failures of fear appeals.

We call our theory the Extended Parallel Process Model (EPPM). The EPPM is not really an original theory but rather an integration of all of the previous theoretical perspectives. It takes the best from previous fear appeal and other behavioral change theories and combines them to explain different responses to health threats. In this chapter, we present the EPPM. The rest of this book focuses on developing effective health risk messages according to the principles suggested by the EPPM.

■■ THE OVERALL MODEL

The Extended Parallel Process Model is based on Leventhal's Parallel Process Model. If you remember, this model suggested two distinct processes in response to fear appeals—a danger control process and a fear control process. However, Leventhal's model was criticized for lacking specificity and predictive power (Beck & Frankel, 1981). In developing the Extended Parallel Process Model (EPPM), we returned to Leventhal's work and expanded upon it. We first specified what leads to danger control versus fear control. Then, we identified the underlying mechanisms occurring in each process. Next, we explained when one process would be expected to dominate over the other. Finally, we detailed what outcomes to expect with each process.

Many elements of older fear appeal theories appear in the EPPM because we did not want to reinvent the wheel when we believed that for the most part, these theories were right. At the same time, the EPPM goes beyond these previous models because it presents a holistic view of responses and reactions to fear appeals, that is, both the successes and failures.

In general, the EPPM suggests health risk messages initiate two cognitive appraisals—an appraisal of the threat and an appraisal of the efficacy of the recommended response. Based on these appraisals, one of three outcomes results—no response, a danger control response, or a fear control response (see Figure 3.1).

The first cognitive appraisal is of the threat. Cognitive appraisal is simply another way of saying, "thinking about an issue." Thus, when people are "cognitively appraising the threat," they are simply "thinking about the threat." So, when presented with a health risk, people first think about whether it is relevant to them (e.g., "am I at risk for experiencing this threat"—perceived susceptibility) and whether the threat is significant (e.g., "could I be significantly harmed by this threat?"— perceived severity). If the threat is deemed to be irrelevant and/or trivial, people do not process any further information about the threat. They just ignore it and don't respond to the risk message because they believe the threat doesn't really affect them anyway. Thus, if individuals have *low* perceived susceptibility and/or *low* perceived severity, then they simply do not respond to a risk message.

In contrast, if people "appraise" or think about the threat and believe they are vulnerable to it and/or it could lead to serious harm, then they become fearful and motivated to act. The stronger the threat is perceived to be, the greater the fear and the stronger the motivation to do something about it. At this point, people appraise or think about the efficacy of the recommended response. Depending on the level of efficacy appraised, people perform one of two responses, either a danger control or a fear control response.

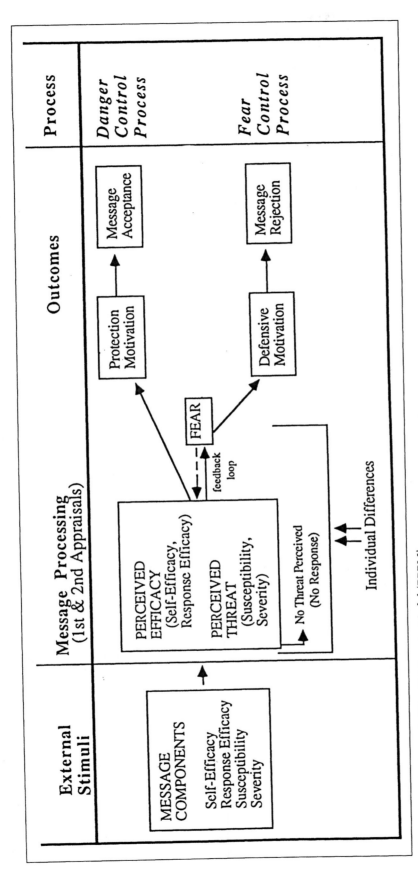

Figure 3.1 The Extended Parallel Process Model (EPPM)

High Perceived Efficacy Conditions
When Perceived Threat is High

If individuals believe they can perform the recommended response (e.g., "It's easy for me to wear my seatbelt each time I'm in the car"—high perceived self-efficacy), and they believe the recommended response works in averting the threat (e.g., "I know that wearing my seatbelt protects me if I'm in an accident"—high perceived response efficacy), their heightened perceptions of threat and efficacy motivate them to control the danger. When individuals control the danger, they take actions to protect themselves against it (protection motivation). Usually, the actions taken are recommended in the message. Thus, a health risk message is seen as successful when people control the danger because people are making the changes necessary to protect themselves against the threat. Danger control responses are usually changes in attitude, intention, and behavior in line with the message's recommendations. Danger control responses have been the focus of nearly all fear appeal work prior to ours (Rippetoe & Rogers, 1987, is a notable exception).

Low Perceived Efficacy Conditions
When Perceived Threat is High

If individuals doubt their ability to perform the recommended response (e.g., "I don't think I can quit smoking; it's too hard"—low perceived self-efficacy) and/or they doubt whether the recommended response really averts the threat (e.g., "Even if I did quit smoking it's probably too late for me; I probably already have pre-cancerous cells"—low perceived response efficacy), they believe there's no use in controlling the danger. They turn their attention instead to controlling their fear (defensive motivation). Individuals usually use psychological defense strategies to control their fears, such as defensive avoidance, denial, or reactance.

Defensive avoidance occurs when people block further thoughts or feelings about a given health threat. It is a type of perceptual defense (see Witte, 1994, for full discussion). When defensive avoidance occurs, individuals distort or ignore incoming information about a threat. Selective attention and exposure, which occur when people avoid exposing themselves to information about the threat, may result. For example, individuals with high threat/low efficacy perceptions toward HIV/AIDS may flip the television channel or skip a magazine article on HIV/AIDS to avoid dealing with the subject.

Denial is when people flat-out refuse to believe they could experience the health threat. They might believe that "other" people may experience the health threat but they are protected in some magical way. Beliefs like "God is protecting me, I have special immune properties," or "only good things happen to me," are examples of beliefs people list when they engage in denial.

When reactance occurs, individuals often say the risk message or the source of the risk message is trying to manipulate them. This perceived manipulation prompts individuals to either reject the message outright or to become angry about the whole issue. Thus, instead of controlling the danger, they control their fear by thinking that "the government" or "doctors" (or whoever the source of the message is) are trying to manipulate them into acting in a certain way. In a study conducted on radon awareness, for example, it was found that when individuals felt threatened by risks of radon exposure and believed there was little they could do to prevent harm from this exposure (i.e., high perceived threat/low perceived efficacy), the study participants began to question whether the whole issue of radon was a government plot. Subsequently, they began to convince themselves that radon was probably made up to scare people (Witte, Berkowitz, Lillie, Cameron, Lapinski, & Liu, 1998). Thus, these individuals controlled their fear about the threat of radon by convincing themselves that the whole issue wasn't real; it was just a government plot.

The Relationship Between Threat and Efficacy

It is important to note that perceived threat motivates action—any kind of action. The stronger the threat is perceived to be, then the greater the fear aroused and the stronger the motivation to act. Perceived efficacy determines the nature of this action, whether people control the danger or control their fear. People tend to evaluate the efficacy of the recommended response in light of the strength of the perceived threat to determine the ease, feasibility, and practicality of performing the recommended response. As long as perceived efficacy is stronger than perceived threat, individuals engage in danger control processes. Thus, high perceived efficacy (i.e., people feel able to perform an effective recommended response) coupled with high perceived threat (i.e., people believe they are vulnerable to a significant threat) promotes protection motivation and danger control responses. As a result, people think carefully about the recommended responses advocated in a persuasive message and adopt those behaviors to control the danger (e.g., "I know that if my partner uses a condom every time we have sex, we can protect each other from AIDS. I'm going to keep some in my purse"). Fear has a somewhat tangential role in danger control processes. Although fear is not directly related to danger control responses such as attitude, intention, or behavior change, it can be indirectly related when it causes individuals to upgrade their estimates of a perceived threat.

At some critical point, however, perceptions of threat may begin to exceed perceptions of efficacy. For example, people may start doubting that condoms really prevent HIV infection and/or they may doubt their ability to bring up the issue of condoms with a sexual partner. At this critical point, where perceived threat begins to exceed perceived efficacy, people shift into fear control processes (bypassing all thoughts about threat and efficacy), and focus on managing their fear, instead of managing the danger.

People engage in fear control processes when they do not think they can adopt an effective response to avert a serious and relevant threat because the response is too hard, too costly, takes too much time, or they think it will not work (i.e., low perceived response and self-efficacy). Thus, low perceived efficacy (i.e., people feel *unable* to perform a response and/or believe the response to be ineffective) coupled with high perceived threat (i.e., people believe they are vulnerable to a significant threat) promotes defensive motivation and fear control responses. As a result, people focus on how frightened they feel and try to eliminate their fear through denial (e.g., "I'm not at risk for AIDS; I'm special"), defensive avoidance (e.g., "This is just too scary; I'm simply not going to think about it"), or reactance (e.g., "They're just trying to manipulate me; I'm going to ignore them"). Fear plays a critical role in fear control processes as it is the direct cause of defensive avoidance, reactance, and other fear control responses. Cognition or thoughts about the recommended response play little part in fear control processes because people have given up thinking about the danger and are attempting instead to control their fear.

Overall, the EPPM suggests that individuals implicitly weigh perceived threat against perceived efficacy in a multiplicative manner in their cognitive appraisal. Therefore, an interaction between threat and efficacy would be expected. The *critical point,* when perceived threat exceeds perceived efficacy, is when the previously dominant danger control processes take second place to fear control processes. This critical point is an important concept in the development of effective health risk messages and is discussed further in Chapter 6.

Individual Differences

Individual differences, such as worldviews (i.e., individualism/collectivism), trait variables (e.g., locus of control, anxiety, sensation seeking), or prior experiences do not appear to directly influence outcomes (e.g., attitudes, intentions, behaviors, defensive avoidance, reactance, etc.), according to the EPPM. Instead, individual differences are posited to influence perceptions of threat and efficacy only, and then these perceptions influence outcomes. For example, individuals who are highly anxious by nature are likely to perceive threats and the efficacy of a recommended response differently than individuals who have low trait anxiety by nature. High- and low-anxiety individuals are likely to combine their perceptions of threat and efficacy in different manners and may end up undergoing different parallel processes. For example, highly anxious people tend to see threats as worse than they really are and recommended responses as more difficult to undertake than they really are. Thus, highly anxious people may be more likely to reach the critical point where perceived threat exceeds perceived efficacy (resulting in fear control processes) sooner than low-anxiety people. Thus, the EPPM suggests that individual differences *indirectly* influence outcomes, as mediated by perceptions of threat and efficacy.

Summary

Overall, the EPPM suggests that two appraisal processes (i.e., threat appraisal and efficacy appraisal) lead to one of three outcomes:

   a. no response when perceived threat is low,
   b. primarily cognitive danger control processes leading to acceptance of fear-arousing messages when perceived threat and perceived efficacy are high, and
   c. primarily emotional fear control processes leading to rejection of fear-arousing messages when perceived threat is high but perceived efficacy is low.

Perceived threat determines the strength or how much of a response there is to a risk message, whereas perceived efficacy determines the nature of the response—whether a risk message induces danger control or fear control processes. Fear directly causes fear control responses but can indirectly influence danger control responses when mediated by perceptions of threat. Individual differences can indirectly influence outcomes when they influence perceptions of threat and efficacy. Table 3.1 defines important terms from the EPPM.

Table 3.1   Definitions of Important Concepts from the EPPM (see also Table 2.1).

Danger Control	A cognitive process eliciting protection motivation that occurs when one believes s/he is able to effectively avert a significant and relevant threat through self-protective changes. When in danger control, people think of strategies to avert a threat.
Danger Control Responses	Belief, attitude, intention, and behavior changes in accordance with a message's recommendations.
Fear Control	An emotional process eliciting defensive motivation that occurs when people are faced with a significant and relevant threat but believe themselves to be unable to perform a recommended response and/or they believe the response to be ineffective. The high levels of fear caused by this condition produce defensive motivation resulting in coping responses that reduce fear and prevent danger control responses from occurring.
Fear Control Responses	Coping responses that diminish fear such as defensive avoidance, denial, and reactance (including issue/message derogation and perceived manipulative intent).
Critical Point	The point where perceptions of threat begin to exceed perceptions of efficacy, causing fear control processes to begin dominating over danger control processes.

THE DEPICTION OF THE MODEL ■■

Figure 3.1 illustrates the EPPM. Although it is difficult to graphically present the model because of the complex relationships between threat, efficacy, and fear, Figure 3.1 gives a rough approximation of how danger control and fear control processes operate. Briefly, health risk messages act as external stimuli to prompt some sort of message processing. First, threat is appraised. If the threat is believed to be relevant and serious, then efficacy is appraised. If no threat is perceived, then there is no response to the health risk message. If perceived threat is high, then individuals are motivated to act. If individuals have high levels of perceived efficacy, then they are motivated to protect themselves (i.e., protection motivation), and they accept the risk message's recommendations and perform the necessary self-protective behaviors. If perceived efficacy is low, then individuals become so fearful, they must cope with and control their fear. Thus, defensive mechanisms are elicited under high threat/low efficacy conditions (i.e., defensive motivation), and individuals reject the message and turn instead to fear control strategies such as defensive avoidance, denial, or reactance. Sometimes, it is reasonable and even adaptive to control one's fear. For example, if one is faced with a terrible threat with little hope of averting it, it is psychologically adaptive to control one's fear and defensively avoid the threat (i.e., avoid thinking about or worrying about the threat). Notice that the top portion of the model, the danger control processes, is really the original Protection Motivation Theory with self-efficacy added. Thus, PMT is incorporated into the EPPM. The fear control side of the model incorporates some of Hovland, Janis, and Kelly's (1953) original ideas from the Fear-as-Acquired Drive Model. Although elements of these models are incorporated into the EPPM, the EPPM expands on these previous theories in important ways.

COMPARISONS WITH OTHER MODELS ■■

The EPPM differs from other risk message models in four important ways. First, in previous fear appeal models, no distinction was made as to how people initially process risk messages. It was assumed people exposed to a risk message would process it all at once. For example, in PMT, the four components of a risk message are proposed to automatically induce four corresponding cognitive mediators, specifically, susceptibility, severity, response efficacy, and self-efficacy. In contrast, the EPPM suggests that two appraisals operate sequentially. First, the threat appraisal must produce a certain threshold level of perceived threat before people even consider the recommended response in the efficacy appraisal. Once the threshold is reached, then the second appraisal of the efficacy of the recommended response occurs. Threat determines how strongly individuals respond to risk messages (i.e., how much behavioral change or how much defensive avoidance), and efficacy determines which responses occur (i.e., either danger control or fear control responses).

Second, the EPPM suggests that perceived threat and fear are conceptually distinct. Previous studies interchangeably used the terms "threat" and "fear" as synonyms. However, research on the EPPM suggests that although highly correlated, they are distinct concepts resulting in fundamentally different outcomes (see Table 2.1 in Chapter 2). Specifically, the EPPM suggests that fear directly causes fear control responses and is unrelated to danger control responses. Cognitions or thoughts about the threat and especially, about the recommended response, directly cause danger control responses. Thus, fear dominates in the primarily emotional fear control processes and thoughts about the threat and the efficacy of the recommended responses dominate in the primarily cognitive danger control processes.

Third, prior to the development of the EPPM, most health risk message researchers measured only attitude, intention, and behavior changes. They did not measure other outcomes that might interfere with these changes. Health risk messages can and do produce outcomes other than attitude, intention, and behavior changes. The EPPM suggests that in addition to measuring danger control responses, researchers should measure fear control responses such as defensive avoidance, denial, or reactance.

Fourth, the EPPM broadens the scope of outcomes produced by health risk messages. Previous health risk message research focused on two outcomes in response to health risk messages—message success, defined as adoption of recommended attitudes or behaviors, and message failure, defined as non-adoption of recommended attitudes or behaviors. Previous research did not distinguish *why* health risk messages failed. The EPPM suggests two reasons for health risk message failure: (a) the message failed to produce any response; people simply did not process it; or (b) the message produced fear control outcomes such as defensive avoidance, denial, or reactance. When a campaign fails, it is critical to determine whether it was because there was no response to the messages or whether the campaign prompted fear control responses. If the former is true, then future campaign messages need to emphasize people's susceptibility to the threat and the severity of the threat. Stronger motivation is needed to promote action. If the latter is true, then a potentially dangerous situation has developed. Once fear control processes are initiated, they are extremely difficult to reverse. For example, if you are defensively avoiding your risk of skin cancer, then you avoid listening to or reading about skin cancer and you continue to put yourself in danger. Special health risk messages need to be developed to break through these psychological defense mechanisms when fear control responses occur.

CHAPTER 3

▪▪ RESEARCH ON THE EPPM

The EPPM has been tested with a variety of research methods including experiments, surveys, focus groups, and content analyses. Tractor safety, skin cancer, HIV/AIDS prevention, dental hygiene, genital warts, radon awareness, violence prevention, and electromagnetic fields are some of the topics in EPPM studies. Similarly, EPPM studies have focused on many different populations, including juvenile delinquents, high school students, Kenyan prostitutes, college students, African-American homeowners, farmers, gun owners, and the general public. Across these diverse topics and populations, relatively consistent results have emerged. Namely, threat appears to interact with efficacy such that high threat/high efficacy messages promote danger control processes leading to acceptance of the message's recommendations. High threat/low efficacy messages promote fear control processes leading to rejection of the message's recommendations and performance of various psychological defenses. However, exceptions to the general pattern of findings have also occurred. Therefore, much more research is needed before we can conclusively say that the EPPM is an accurate health risk message model. However, given the current evidence, it offers fairly clear advice on how to develop health risk messages that work and how to avoid developing health risk messages that don't work.[1]

NOTE ▪▪

1. For more information on the EPPM, please see Witte, K. (1998), Fear as Motivator, Fear as Inhibitor: Using the Extended Parallel Process Models to Explain Fear Appeal Successes and Failures (pp. 423-450), in P. A. Andersen & L. K. Guerrero (Eds.), *The Handbook of Communication and Emotion: Research, Theory, Applications, and Contexts.* Academic Press.

4

Useful Concepts from Other Theories

M any other theoretical approaches to health behavior change exist. This chapter examines concepts from the most popular approaches and illustrates how they can be used to develop health risk messages. You'll notice that the variables across many of these models are similar. In fact, the majority of health behavior change models focus on the variables of threat, efficacy, and barriers. In addition to the fear appeal theories outlined previously, the four most common persuasive message theories are:

a. the Health Belief Model,
b. the Theory of Reasoned Action,
c. Social Cognitive Theory, and
d. the Elaboration Likelihood Model.

In addition to these four theoretical models are two approaches or strategies often used in health risk message development—the Stages of Change Model (or Transtheoretical Model) and Social Marketing. The difference between theories and approaches is that theories *explain* how variables work together to influence health behaviors and approaches *describe* different steps to increase the persuasiveness of a health risk message. Each of these perspectives is discussed in turn in this chapter.

THE HEALTH BELIEF MODEL ■■

The Health Belief Model (HBM) (Janz & Becker, 1984; Rosenstock, 1974) is one of the most commonly used models of health behavior change and is probably the most frequently taught model in health intervention courses. Many health professionals have used it to guide the development of intervention and campaign efforts, and its influence on health communication research is enormous. It was developed as an overarching framework for promoting preventive behaviors (such as immunizations) by a group of social psychologists in the early 1950s (Janz & Becker, 1984). Briefly, the HBM suggests that preventive health behavior is influenced by five factors:

    a. perceived barriers to performing the recommended response;
    b. perceived benefits of performing the recommended response;
    c. perceived susceptibility to a health threat;
    d. perceived severity of a health threat; and
    e. cues to action (see Figure 4.1).

The HBM suggests that individuals weigh the potential benefits of the recommended response against the psychological, physical, and financial costs of the action (the barriers) when deciding to act. For example, a nurse may realize the benefit of having up-to-date medical information (a recommended action) but may lack access, the skills, or even the transportation needed to get to a library. In this case, lack of access, lack of needed skills, and lack of transportation all act as barriers. These barriers outweigh any benefits of the information, and the nurse probably would not seek it out. Similarly, the HBM suggests that individuals evaluate the severity of a threat and whether they are really susceptible. Rosenstock (1974) has noted that the combination of perceived susceptibility and severity provides the motivation for action, and the comparison of perceived benefits to perceived barriers provides the means or pathway to action. Thus, the stronger the perceptions of severity, susceptibility, and benefits, and the weaker the perception of barriers are, the greater is the likelihood that health-protective actions would be taken. That is, if you feel susceptible to a terrible disease, believe a vaccination can protect you (strong benefit), and can get the shot free of charge (low barrier), then you probably will get it.

Demographics and prior experiences are said to affect the four variables just described (i.e., perceived susceptibility, severity, benefits, and barriers) as well as "cues to action." Cues to action can be anything that prompts one to think about a health issue or act on it. Internal cues such as a cough might prompt a smoker to have a lung X-ray. External cues such as a television commercial might prompt a woman to do a breast self-examination. Cues are suggested to increase perceptions of susceptibility and severity, and in turn, trigger decision making in which perceived barriers and benefits are weighed against each other. For example, if you read a magazine article about skin cancer, it may act as an external cue that increases your perception of susceptibility to the disease and the severity of the disease. If your perceptions of susceptibility and severity are increased, you may be motivated to act. As a result, you may compare the benefits of wearing sunscreen (the recommended action) against the barriers to wearing sunscreen. Most likely you will weigh the benefits of being protected against skin cancer against the barriers of social pressures of being pale-skinned and greasy. Depending on the strength of the barriers, you may or may not adopt the recommended action of wearing sunscreen.

The HBM has been empirically tested as the basis for many campaigns including bicycle helmet use (Witte, Stokols, Ituarte, Schneider, 1993; see Figure 4.2), vaccination for infectious diseases (Larson, Bergman, 1982), adolescent fertility control (Eisen, Zellman, & McAlister, 1985), and risky sexual practices (Vanlandingham, Suprasert, Grandjean, & Sittitrai, 1995). Witte, Stokels, Ituarte, and Schneider (1993) used the graphics shown in Figure 4.2 to show the benefits of wearing bike helmets. Overall, perceived barriers have been the strongest predictor of whether individuals engage in

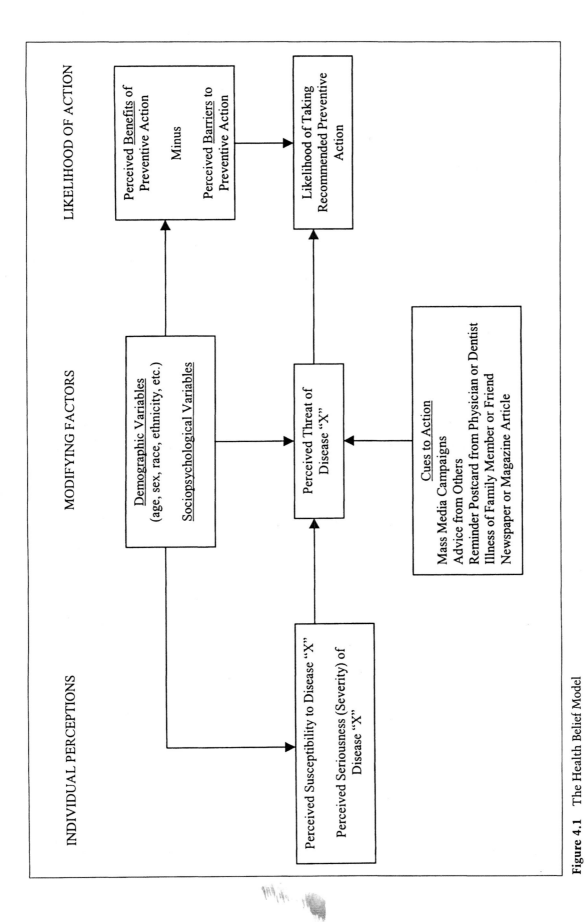

INDIVIDUAL PERCEPTIONS   **MODIFYING FACTORS**   **LIKELIHOOD OF ACTION**

Perceived <u>Benefits</u> of Preventive Action

Minus

Perceived <u>Barriers</u> to Preventive Action

Likelihood of Taking Recommended Preventive Action

<u>Demographic Variables</u> (age, sex, race, ethnicity, etc.)

<u>Sociopsychological Variables</u>

Perceived Threat of Disease "X"

<u>Cues to Action</u>
Mass Media Campaigns
Advice from Others
Reminder Postcard from Physician or Dentist
Illness of Family Member or Friend
Newspaper or Magazine Article

Perceived Susceptibility to Disease "X"

Perceived Seriousness (Severity) of Disease "X"

CHAPTER 4

Figure 4.1 The Health Belief Model

SOURCE: Reprinted from *Health Education & Behavior, 11*(1)(1984) with permission of Sage Publications, Inc.

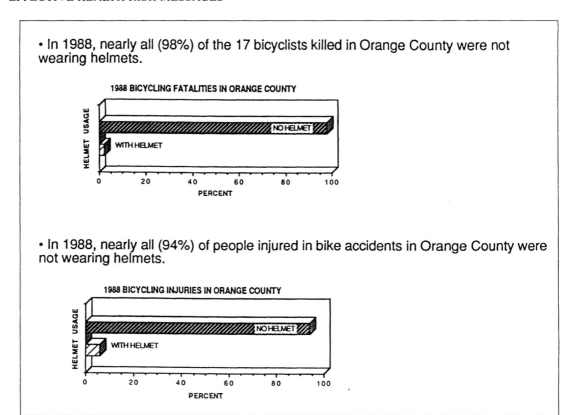

Figure 4.2 Facts about bike helmets

health-protective behaviors, followed by perceived susceptibility (Janz & Becker, 1984). Janz and Becker (1984) found that perceived severity was the weakest predictor across studies using the HBM. Thus, it is important to assess perceived barriers to recommended actions. We are of the opinion that perceived barriers are strongly related to perceived self-efficacy (and may even be the converse of high self-efficacy). For example, barriers, such as financial costs, psychological costs, resource costs, and so on, all inhibit one's perceived ability to perform the recommended response. Thus, barriers seem to be the explanatory variable for low self-efficacy perceptions (i.e., why don't you feel able to perform the recommended response? Because of barriers X, Y, and Z). Regardless of whether you think barriers are distinct from self-efficacy, the variable should be addressed in your health risk message. This issue is addressed in the next chapter.

In sum, the HBM may be viewed as the grandmother of most modern health education theories. As such, its variables and principles can be seen in many health risk message models.

▊▊ THE THEORY OF REASONED ACTION

Often messages created for outreach efforts are based on intuitive appeal, rather than sound methodology (Fishbein & Ajzen, 1981). Even if a theory is used to develop messages, campaigners tend to use the variables in the theory as guidelines for material to include without considering the actual content or words in a message. For example, campaign designers might address the severity of a threat and the audience's susceptibility to that threat—the theoretical variables—in a message, but the actual words or images used to address these variables are not systematically chosen. Fishbein and Ajzen (1981) go so far as to conclude that "the general neglect of the information contained in a message and its relation to the dependent variable is probably the most serious problem in communication and persuasion research" (p. 359).

Fishbein and Ajzen (1975; 1981) suggest specific message construction and evaluation techniques based on their Theory of Reasoned Action (TRA). In TRA, Fishbein and Ajzen (1975) propose that a person's behavior is predicted by intentions, which, in turn, are predicted by attitudes toward the behavior *and* subjective norms. Attitudes are predicted by behavioral beliefs and evaluations of those beliefs. Subjective norms are predicted by normative beliefs and the motivation to comply with those normative beliefs. Fishbein and Ajzen (1975) state that two sets of beliefs must be altered prior to behavior change:

1. Beliefs about the consequences of performing a certain behavior and the evaluation of those consequences (attitude)

2. Beliefs about what other people or referents think about the behavior to be performed and the motivation to comply with those referents (subjective norm)

Only when a message targets the salient beliefs of these variables do attitudes and subjective norms, and subsequently, behavioral intentions and behavior, change (see Figure 4.3). Salient beliefs are those first five to seven beliefs that come to mind when you think about an issue.

The first step to using TRA is to analyze an audience's beliefs about specific behaviors. Say you wish to promote bicycle helmets to prevent head injuries in accidents. You first need to determine attitudes toward wearing bicycle helmets and the subjective norm toward wearing bicycle helmets. Let's start with attitudes. First, you would survey for salient beliefs about the consequences of wearing a bicycle helmet. What are people's beliefs about wearing bicycle helmets? What are the advantages and disadvantages to wearing helmets? Second, you ask individuals to give a rating as to the strength of each salient belief. Do you strongly believe that wearing a bicycle helmet messes up your hair or do you just slightly believe that it messes up your hair? Third, you ask individuals to evaluate each belief *separately from the attitude object*. In our case, the attitude object is bicycle helmets (i.e., we're determining attitudes toward bicycle helmets). So, you want to find out individuals' evaluations of each belief. For example, anything that "messes up my hair" (the belief related to the attitude object of wearing a bicycle helmet) is bad. Anything that "protects against head injuries" (the belief) is good. Anything that "costs a lot of money" is bad. And, so on. Now, you multiply each belief strength by each evaluation and then sum the products. The total sum gives you the overall attitude toward wearing bicycle helmets.

It is very important to gather all salient beliefs on a given attitude object or recommended response. If you gathered only one belief and targeted it in a persuasive message, it is unlikely the overall attitude toward the recommended response would change because these other beliefs have remained strong. Therefore, you need to change the entire set of underlying beliefs toward the recommended response so that the attitude shifts.

Table 4.1 indicates a college student's hypothetical attitude toward wearing bicycle helmets. Recall that attitudes are comprised of one's beliefs toward the attitude object

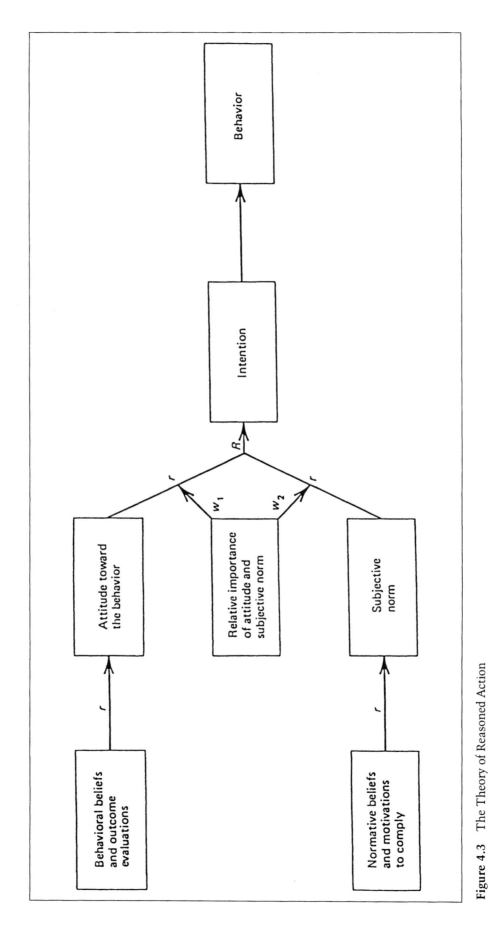

Figure 4.3 The Theory of Reasoned Action

SOURCE: From *Understanding Attitudes and Predicting Social Behavior* by Ajzen & Fishbein, © 1980. Reprinted by permission of Prentice-Hall, Inc., Upper Saddle River, NJ.

Table 4.1 Hypothetical Attitude Toward Wearing a Bicycle Helmet

Salient Beliefs	Strength of Beliefs	Evaluation of Beliefs	Product
1. "messes up my hair"	.60	−3	−1.80
2. "costs a lot"	.50	−2	−1.00
3. "protects against head injury"	.70	3	2.10
Total Attitude Toward Wearing a Bicycle Helmet (sum)			−0.70

(in this case bicycle helmets) multiplied by the evaluation of the individual beliefs (whether they are good or bad). This person believes that bicycle helmets mess up one's hair, cost a lot, and protect against injury. These are his salient beliefs about wearing bicycle helmets. The strength of these beliefs (ranging from .00 to 1.00) is indicated in the second column and the evaluation of these attributes is indicated in the third column, ranging from -3 (unfavorable) to +3 (favorable). These belief strengths and evaluations are multiplied individually and then summed to create the overall attitude toward wearing bicycle helmets. For example, this person has a moderately strong belief that wearing bicycle helmets messes up hair (.60) and anything that messes up hair is evaluated unfavorably (-3). In addition, he believes somewhat that bicycle helmets cost a lot (.5), and anything that costs a lot is evaluated unfavorably, too (-2). Finally, he strongly believes that bicycle helmets protect against injury (.70) and anything that protects against injury is evaluated favorably (+3). The sum of these products indicates that this person's predominant attitude toward wearing bicycle helmets is somewhat negative at -0.70.

Subjective norm is determined in a similar manner. First, you determine who the salient referents—or important others—are with reference to wearing bicycle helmets. For example, what person or group of persons has an impact on your decision to wear or not wear a bicycle helmet? Second, you find out whether your target audience thinks their salient referent thinks performing the recommended behavior is good or bad (the normative belief). Notice, you do not determine what salient referents really think. Rather, you determine what target audience members *think* their salient referents think. Third, you assess target audience members' motivation to comply with each referent. Finally, you multiply normative belief by motivation to comply and sum the products to yield an overall subjective norm. Table 4.2 gives a hypothetical example of a college student's subjective norm toward wearing bicycle helmets. His salient referents (those people most important to him) with respect to wearing bicycle helmets are his girlfriend, his best friend, his parents, and his favorite professor (who is of course, his health risk message professor). His normative beliefs reflect what *he* thinks each of these specific referents think about his wearing a bicycle helmet (ranging from -3 [should not use] to +3 [should use]).

This person thinks his girlfriend and best friend have slightly negative beliefs toward him wearing a bicycle helmet (-1) and that his parents and favorite professor have slightly positive beliefs toward him wearing a bicycle helmet (+1). His motivation to comply with each referent is indicated on a scale from 0 (not at all) to 3 (strongly). This person is strongly motivated to comply with his girlfriend (3) and his best friend (3) but

Table 4.2   Hypothetical Subjective Norm Toward Wearing Bicycle Helmets

Salient Referents	Normative Belief	Motivation to Comply	Product
1. Girlfriend	−1	3	−3
2. Best friend	−1	3	−3
3. Parents	+1	1	1
4. Favorite Professor	+1	1	1
Total Subjective Norm Toward Wearing Bicycle Helmets			−4

not with his parents (1) or favorite professor (1). In each case, the normative belief and the motivation to comply is multiplied to yield a product and the sum of these products is the subjective norm. This person's overall subjective norm toward wearing bicycle helmets is moderately negative.

The attitude and subjective norms are sometimes weighted according to their importance, and then combined, to influence intentions, which then influence behaviors. Overall, this college student's scores suggest that he would not wear bicycle helmets because both his attitude and subjective norm were negative toward his doing so. A campaign directly targeting his negative salient beliefs regarding wearing bicycle helmets would be appropriate here. For example, this person believes that bicycle helmets cost a lot. To counteract this salient belief, campaigners can offer coupons to lower the cost and can suggest "for the price of two meals out you can save your skull," or "you can buy a helmet for less than half the cost of a visit to the doctor or 1/8th the cost of a visit to the emergency room." These statements suggest that helmets are affordable and within one's everyday budget.

Overall, TRA is one of the few theories to offer a systematic approach to the construction of the content of health risk messages. It has been applied to a number of health-related behaviors, including the impact of health risk messages about tap water (Griffin, Neuwirth, & Dunwoody, 1995), sexual practices and AIDS related-behaviors (Fishbein & Middlestadt, 1989; Fishbein, Middlestadt, & Hitchcock, 1991; Vanlandingham, Suprasert, Grandjean, & Sittirai, 1995), childbearing intentions (Crawford & Boyer, 1985), testicular cancer prevention (Brubaker & Wickersham, 1990), exercise in schoolchildren (Ferguson, Yesalis, Pomrehn, & Kirkpatrick, 1989), alcoholism (Fishbein, Ajzen, & McArdle, 1980), cigarette smoking (Norman & Tedeschi, 1989), violence prevention (Roberto, Meyer, Boster, & Story, 2000), and many others.

▓▓ SOCIAL-COGNITIVE THEORY

Albert Bandura's Social Cognitive Theory (sometimes called Social Learning Theory) has been used in a wide variety of health intervention efforts (see Figure 4.4). It was used in the Stanford 5-Cities project to prevent heart disease and, more recently, has been used in several AIDS-prevention projects. The focus of the theory is *perceived self-efficacy*. Self-efficacy is defined as "people's beliefs that they can exert control over their motivation and behavior and over their social environment" (Bandura, 1989, p. 128). As in fear appeals, perceived self-efficacy is what you believe about your ability to perform a

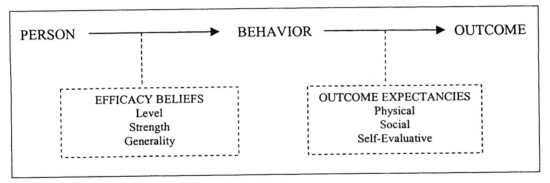

Figure 4.4 Social Cognitive Theory

SOURCE: Self-efficacy: Toward a unifying theory of behavioral change, by A. Bandura. *Psychological Review*, *84*, 191-215. (1977). Copyright © 1977 by the American Psychological Association. Reprinted with permission.

certain action (your perceived self-effectiveness). Bandura (1977) views self-efficacy as the driving force of human behavior. "Efficacy expectations are a major determinant of people's choice of activities, how much effort they will expend, and of how long they will sustain effort in dealing with stressful situations" (Bandura, 1977, p. 194).

Another important construct in Bandura's theory is *outcome expectations*. Outcome expectations (similar to response efficacy in fear appeals) refer to an individual's belief that a certain behavior leads to a certain outcome. For example, "I believe if I wear a bicycle helmet I will not be injured in an accident" is an outcome expectation. It's what you think will happen if you take a certain action. Outcome expectations are different from efficacy expectations in that the latter is your belief concerning whether you can "successfully execute the behavior required to produce the outcomes" (Bandura, 1977, p. 193). For example, even if outcome expectations are high, efficacy expectations can be low, similar to the way response efficacy can be high but self-efficacy can be low (i.e., "I believe that eating a low fat diet is good for my health [outcome expectations/response efficacy] but I'm just not able to eat a low-fat diet [self-efficacy]). In short, according to social cognitive theory, a person can believe certain actions lead to particular outcomes (outcome expectations), but this individual may doubt his or her ability to perform the action (efficacy expectations). According to Bandura (1977), only when efficacy expectations are high can people perform certain behaviors. Efficacy expectations can vary on dimensions of magnitude (level of difficulty of task; people may have different efficacy expectations for simple tasks than for difficult tasks), generality (specific to general), and strength (weak to strong) (Bandura, 1977).

Bandura (1977) states that an individual's self-efficacy perceptions are developed from four sources of information: performance accomplishments, physiological states, verbal persuasion, and vicarious experience. Participant modeling or performance desensitization are examples of performance accomplishments. That is, you actually practice the recommended behavior (e.g., practice breast or testicular self-examination). Suggestion, exhortation, and self-instruction are what constitute verbal persuasion (e.g., commercials or pamphlets). Vicarious experience stems from live or symbolic modeling (e.g., watching other people do breast or testicular self-examination). Finally, physiological or emotional arousal comes from relaxation, biofeedback, and symbolic desensitization or exposure. Bandura's Social Cognitive Theory is well-integrated into the Extended Parallel Process Model and Protection Motivation Theory. Therefore, although the terminology may sound slightly different, the concepts should be familiar.

◫ ELABORATION LIKELIHOOD MODEL

The Elaboration Likelihood Model (ELM; Petty & Cacioppo, 1986) focuses on how information is processed and the relationship between information processing and behavior change (see Figure 4.5). Given the same message, two people may process the information in very different ways because of their cultural background, prior experiences, personalities, mood states, and so on, and come up with very different decisions regarding whether to engage in a behavior or not. The Elaboration Likelihood Model (Petty & Cacioppo, 1986) argues that individuals process messages via either the peripheral route or the central route (see also the Systematic-Heuristic model for a similar but conceptually distinct model in Chaiken, 1980, 1987). When people process a message *peripherally*, they do not thoughtfully consider the arguments in the message and use various cues like attractiveness, reputation, credibility, and so on, to guide their decision whether to perform a behavior. When people have little interest, ability, and/or motivation to think about a message, they tend to process it peripherally. For example, when people process a message peripherally, they use simple associations or heuristics (i.e., mental models) to make a decision (e.g., "If my dentist uses Crest toothpaste, I should too"; this mental model says that if an expert uses a product, it must be good).

Alternatively, when people have the motivation and ability to think about a topic, they process the message *centrally* by carefully listening to and evaluating the content of the message (Petty & Cacioppo, 1986). Because carefully thinking about a message's arguments or content takes work, messages are centrally processed only when the individual is motivated to do so because (a) they are very important and relevant to a person, and (b) when an individual has the intellectual or technical ability to process a message centrally. For example, you could give an individual lots of technical information about buying a car. The individual still would process it all peripherally if he doesn't know anything about cars and is not *able* to process information about cylinders, horsepower, transmissions, and similar data centrally. This individual is more likely to buy a car based on cues from his friends. For example, his mental model might be exemplified by, "my friends own Jeeps and like them, so they must be good."

Overall, according to the Elaboration Likelihood Model, people must be motivated *and* able to process a message centrally. If people are unable *and/or* not motivated to process a message, then they will process it peripherally. If at all possible, you want to promote central processing because processing via this route leads to long-term and stable change. When you've thought about an issue and made a decision to perform a recommended behavior, you're more committed to really doing it. When you make a decision via the peripheral route (e.g., based on credibility, attractiveness, heuristics), it's easy to change decisions because you're not committed to a particular action. For example, if your favorite celebrity all of a sudden switches from drinking Coke to drinking Pepsi, then you may switch from Coke to Pepsi yourself (at least, that's what the advertisers hope). The ELM has not been used much in the health education and behavior change literature, but it has been used extensively in the advertising, marketing, and persuasion literatures.

◫ STAGES OF CHANGE MODEL

One of a number of stage models of behavior change, the Transtheoretical Model allows practitioners to determine which stage most of their target audience is in with respect to

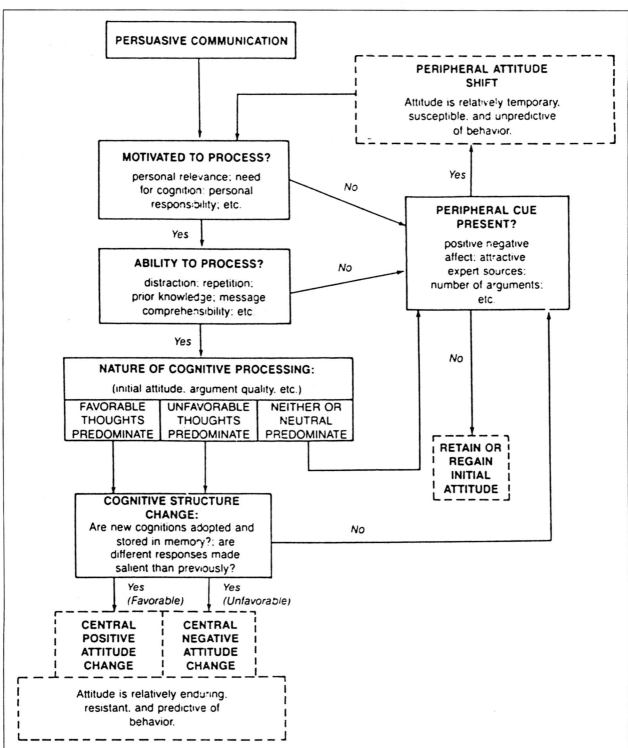

Figure 4.5 Flowchart of the Elaboration Likelihood Model

SOURCE: From *Communication and Persuasion: Central and Peripheral Routes to Attitude Change* by Richard E. Petty and John T. Cacioppo (1986). Reprinted with permission of Springer-Verlag New York, Inc.

CHAPTER 4

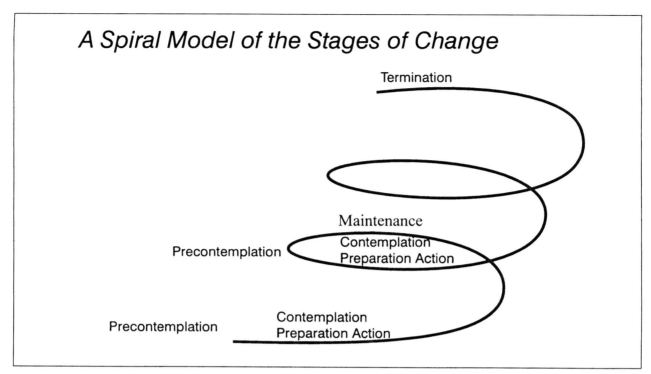

Figure 4.6. A Spiral Model of the Stages of Change

SOURCE: In search of How People Change: Applications to Addictive Behaviors, by J. O. Prochaska, C. C. DiClementes & J. C. Norcross. *American Psychologist, 47*, 1102-1114. (1992). Copyright © 1992 by the American Psychological Association. Reprinted with permission.

a given behavior (DiClemente & Prochaska, 1985). The idea behind the Stages of Change Model (SOC) is to first categorize people according to their stage of "readiness" with respect to the recommended response, and then develop messages that move them from one stage to another (see Figure 4.6). The different stages range from complete unawareness of a health issue to having taken previous action but relapsed into unhealthy behaviors. The Stages of Change Model suggests five stages to the performance of a behavior: Precontemplation, Contemplation, Preparation, Action, and Maintenance. In the *Precontemplative* stage, individuals do not intend to change their behavior because they are completely unaware of the behavioral options available to them. They may not realize they are engaging in a risky behavior, or they may deny their behavior puts them at risk for harm. In the second stage however, this risk becomes apparent to the individual. In the *Contemplation* stage, individuals begin to think about the behavior placing them at risk and to contemplate the need for change. In this stage, for example, an individual recognizes the need for more information. In the third stage, *Preparation*, individuals make a commitment to change and take some action to prepare for the behavioral change, such as taking a class on how to prepare low-fat meals. It is in the *Action* stage that individuals perform the new behavior consistently. In this stage, for example, the individual may regularly eat low-fat foods. In the *Maintenance* stage, the final stage of the SOC model, the new behavior is continued and steps are taken to avoid relapsing into the formerly risky behaviors. For example, a person might continue to learn new low-fat recipes or begin to attend a diet support group.

The SOC model is useful to campaign designers for several reasons. First, individuals in different stages exhibit distinct behavioral characteristics (Weinstein, 1988). Thus, researchers can effectively analyze and segment a target audience according to their different stages of readiness for change. Then, practitioners can strategically design messages to move individuals through the stages (Maibach & Cotton, 1995). For example, if a campaign to promote a new service is needed and it has been determined that the majority of the target population is in the Contemplation stage, health educators can design messages to systematically move this audience through the Preparation, Action, and Maintenance stages. Similarly, if most of the target audience is in the Maintenance stage, educators can provide messages that reinforce and support the desired behavior.

The messages used to move people from one stage to the next differ slightly across stages. Specifically, to move people from the Precontemplation to Contemplation stage, messages need to focus on increasing awareness and knowledge about the health threat and recommended response. To move individuals from the Contemplation to Preparation stage, and from the Preparation to Action stage, messages need to be motivational in nature. That is, they need to motivate people to do something to protect themselves. To move people from the Action stage to the Maintenance stage, messages tend to focus on response efficacy and/or self-efficacy issues. For example, messages that move people from initial actions to the Maintenance stage should focus on the specific skills needed to make a new behavior part of their daily routine. They also need to address the reduction or elimination of barriers that may inhibit maintenance of health behaviors. Knowing the stage of your audience with respect to a health behavior enables you to tailor your message.

The Stages of Change Model has been empirically tested with a number of health topics including smoking cessation, sunscreen use, addictive behaviors, pregnancy prevention, and risky sexual behaviors (e.g., Grimley, Riley, Bellis, & Prochaska, 1993; Prochaska, DiClemente, & Norcross, 1992). It offers a useful typology for segmenting the audience into different groups.

SOCIAL MARKETING ■■

Social marketing is a popular approach to developing health risk messages for large-scale campaigns. It addresses issues of design and implementation of campaign messages and features with the goal of making certain social ideas or principles acceptable for a specific target group (Kotler, 1984; Kotler & Roberto, 1989). Social marketing is the application of for-profit marketing techniques to pro-social health and development programs (Meyer & Dearing, 1996). The idea behind social marketing is to "market" the product (i.e., healthy behavior) in the same aggressive manner that an auto dealership might market a Cadillac. To do this, market researchers discover the basic wants, needs, and desires of the target population and then market the product to fit those needs and desires.

There are several steps to social marketing (Kotler & Roberto, 1989). First, the immediate environment in which the campaign takes place is analyzed. Second, marketers research the target population and divide (segment) the audience into distinct groups with common characteristics. Third, campaign objectives and strategies are developed for each audience segment. When developing campaign strategies, four marketing issues or the "Four Ps" are addressed. The Four Ps are product, price, promotion,

Table 4.3 Summary of Health Behavior Change Theories

Theoretical Origin of Variables	Extended Parallel Process Model	Health Belief Model	Theory of Reasoned Action	Social Cognitive Theory	Elaboration Likelihood Model
Stimuli	Fear Appeals (mass media, interpersonal, group messages, etc.)	Cues to Action Internal External	Observation/ Interaction with Peers	Personal Experiences Vicarious Experience Verbal Persuasion Physiological Arousal	Mass Media Messages Interpersonal Interactions
Motivational Variables	Threat (Susceptibility & Severity) Fear	Threat (Susceptibility & Severity)			Involvement
Internal and Environmental Resources	Self-Efficacy Response Efficacy	Benefits Barriers	Attitudes Subjective Norm	Efficacy Expectations Outcome Expectations	Ability to Process a Message
Outcome Variables	Danger Control Responses (Attitudes, Intentions, Behaviors) Fear Control Responses (Defensive Avoidance, Reactance, Denial)	Intentions Behaviors	Intentions Behaviors	Behaviors	Processing Mode (Central or Peripheral) Attitudes

and place. The product is the behavior the target audience must change or adopt. Campaigns have targeted a number of health behaviors as "products" including condom use, contraception, and alcohol and drug-related behaviors. For example, regular exercise, smoking cessation, dietary changes, and stress reduction were promoted in the Stanford Heart Disease Prevention Project (SHDPP) to prevent heart disease. The second "P" in the marketing mix is price, which includes any actual or perceived physical, social, and psychological costs related to adopting recommended responses. For example, the costs of joining SHDPP's Smoker's Challenge included the money and energy expended in accepting the challenge, as well as the psychological costs of giving up smoking. The third component of the marketing mix, promotion, deals with how the product can be represented or packaged to compensate for the costs of adopting the recommended response. The Stanford project attempted to promote the contest by removing or reducing the financial cost of the program to make it more appealing to target audiences (Lefebvre & Flora, 1988). Place is the final component and addresses the availability of information or products with reference to the recommended response. Every attempt was made to increase access to information in the Stanford project. For example, information on how to quit smoking was mailed to each household participating in the study.

Social marketing has achieved widespread adoption and most large-scale campaigns do some market research before implementation. Social marketing allows campaign developers to carefully target their persuasive materials.

■ SUMMARY

We have presented many popular health behavior change theories and approaches in this chapter. When analyzing the health behavior change theories as a whole, it appears that each theory's variables fall into one of four discrete categories: Stimuli, Motivational Variables, Internal and Environmental Resources, and Outcome Variables. Table 4.3 categorizes each theory's variables.

Briefly, Table 4.3 hypothesizes that stimuli trigger the motivation to do something resulting in an appraisal of internal and environmental resources, leading to one or more outcomes. Stimuli include internal or external cues that cause increased awareness of a health threat. Mass media messages, interpersonal interactions, or any other type of communication are likely to act as stimuli for each theory. Motivation refers to an internal drive state that causes one to act. Appraisals of internal and environmental resources refer to the cognitive evaluation of one's inner and outer cues occurring when one is motivated to act. For instance, when individuals are motivated to act, they consider whether they are able to effectively avert a threat and whether the environment can support this action (e.g., self-efficacy, response efficacy, and access issues). Outcomes include mode of processing (central versus peripheral), as well as danger control responses (i.e., attitudes, intentions, behaviors) and fear control responses (i.e., defensive avoidance, reactance, denial). Note that variables can serve multiple functions. For example, prior attitudes help one form an appraisal of the environment and can also act as an outcome.

To combine theories in a campaign, we suggest you choose at least one variable from each of the theoretical categories when developing your campaign. That is, you need to stimulate, motivate, appraise, and focus on an outcome. For example, a stimulus is necessary to prompt awareness of a health issue. A broadcast Public Service Announcement or talk by a peer educator directly to your audience are two means of providing stimuli. You also need to motivate your audience and address internal resources and environmental issues. According to the theories reviewed here, the two main ways to increase motivation are to increase perceived severity of the threat or increase perceived involvement in a health issue. For example, you could motivate your audience by making them feel susceptible to a terrible new strain of flu (increase perceived threat). Conversely, you could also motivate your audience to act by having them serve, for example, as peer educators for underclassman, thereby motivating them to act as examples and adopt a recommended response themselves. Note that often messages that increase perceived susceptibility also increase perceived involvement because both focus on raising the relevancy of a topic to an individual.

To increase perceived internal and environmental resources, you may choose to focus on self-efficacy (i.e., making individuals feel able to perform a recommended response) or barriers in the environment (e.g., providing transportation to clinics or vouchers for immunizations). Finally, you need to choose specific outcomes. Is your objective attitude change? Increased knowledge? Behavior change? Specify outcomes exactly. Addressing these theoretical issues before starting the campaign improves its effectiveness.

Applying the Stages of Change and Social Marketing perspectives to real-life health campaigns is a bit different from applying the health behavior change theories to campaigns. As stated earlier, the Stages of Change and Social Marketing perspectives offer different ways to approach the development of health risk messages. But they are not theories because they do not offer any explanations as to how different variables, such

Table 4.4 Using Social Marketing and Stages of Change Approaches in Campaigns

Social Marketing	Stages of Changes				
	Pre-Contemplation	Contemplation	Preparation	Action	Maintenance
Product	Stimuli Motivation Appraisals Outcomes	Stimuli Motivation Appraisals Outcomes	Stimuli Motivation Appraisals Outcomes	Stimuli Motivation Appraisals Outcomes	Stimuli Motivation Appraisals Outcomes
Price	Stimuli Motivation Appraisals Outcomes	Stimuli Motivation Appraisals Outcomes	Stimuli Motivation Appraisals Outcomes	Stimuli Motivation Appraisals Outcomes	Stimuli Motivation Appraisals Outcomes
Place	Stimuli Motivation Appraisals Outcomes	Stimuli Motivation Appraisals Outcomes	Stimuli Motivation Appraisals Outcomes	Stimuli Motivation Appraisals Outcomes	Stimuli Motivation Appraisals Outcomes
Promotion	Stimuli Motivation Appraisals Outcomes	Stimuli Motivation Appraisals Outcomes	Stimuli Motivation Appraisals Outcomes	Stimuli Motivation Appraisals Outcomes	Stimuli Motivation Appraisals Outcomes
Outcomes	Stimuli Motivation Appraisals Outcomes	Stimuli Motivation Appraisals Outcomes	Stimuli Motivation Appraisals Outcomes	Stimuli Motivation Appraisals Outcomes	Stimuli Motivation Appraisals Outcomes
Demographics/ Psychographics	Stimuli Motivation Appraisals Outcomes	Stimuli Motivation Appraisals Outcomes	Stimuli Motivation Appraisals Outcomes	Stimuli Motivation Appraisals Outcomes	Stimuli Motivation Appraisals Outcomes

as those appearing in Table 4.3, might work together to explain a certain outcome. When utilizing aspects of the Stages of Change or Social Marketing perspectives, it is important to also address each category of theoretical variables (i.e., stimuli, motivational variables, appraisals of environment and resources, outcomes) in a health campaign. For example, if you wish to develop a product (social marketing task) for your Contemplation-stage audience (specific stage of change), then you should find out (a) the best way to reach them (stimulus), (b) the best way to motivate them, (c) their internal and environmental resources, and (d) what their current outcomes are in response to the health threat. The four theoretical variables should be addressed for each social marketing task and for each stage of change (i.e., each cell in Table 4.4). You may also choose to focus on multiple cells in a communication campaign.

This chapter explained prominent health behavior change theories and approaches used in many communication campaigns today. In addition, we presented an overview on how these different theories and approaches might work together if they were combined. In the next chapter, we discuss one way to combine some of these theories and approaches to conduct formative research on a specific health topic.

5

Starting Out the Right Way

Formative Research

---

ow you have the theoretical knowledge needed to go out and develop effective risk messages. So, how do you translate theory into practice for the field? The next few chapters offer step-by-step guidelines on doing just this. In this chapter we explain how to conduct formative research, sometimes called formative evaluation. This research is conducted *prior* to your intervention or study. It's called formative research because the information discovered in this phase helps to form the final product.

Some people skip formative research and directly develop risk messages and interventions. But in our opinion, this up-front work saves work at the tail end (repeat that 50 times!). Honestly, we have found that the more work you put into a project up front, the better it ends up for all involved. Having some up-front knowledge directly from your target audience results in a smoother and more easily run project. It's similar to going on vacation to a foreign country. If you don't do any up-front research, you may be lucky and have a great trip. However, you may pay high prices because all the hotels are booked; there aren't any fun things to do because a hurricane hit last winter and destroyed all the attractions; and lots of mosquitoes are biting(left over from the hurricane floods). If only you had done some formative research. A little bit of formative research can go a long way toward making a project successful. At this point, you may have thought about your target audience and the topics most important to address to them. Other issues to consider up front are the most effective messages, the length of your campaign, methods of data collection and analysis, and perhaps, even specific methods and channels for disseminating your messages.

This chapter is devoted to effective message development. Later chapters focus on data collection, analysis, and dissemination of your messages. However, it's important to think of all these issues early in a systematic plan. This plan helps organize all the elements of your campaign.

◫ SETTING GOALS AND OBJECTIVES: THE CAMPAIGN PLAN

The first step in developing a plan framework is to state the goals of your campaign. A goal is a general statement describing the ultimate impact of your campaign. Imagine, for example, your university has dedicated the next academic year to improving the safety of its student body, and your campaign is focused on bicycle safety. Given this scenario, your goal may be to "increase the bicycling safety of students at Healthy University." Note this goal statement is broad, and as stated, not amenable to precise measurement. It does, however, fit with the university's mission to improve safety and thus should be attained when Healthy U. assesses the overall safety of students at the year's end and finds improvements.

After stating the goal of your campaign, the next step is to specify campaign objectives. Unlike the campaign's goal, which is rather broad and general, objectives should specify (a) expected outcomes, (b) target audiences, and (c) time frames in which the outcomes will occur. Including these three components in an objective ensures the objective can be measured. It is not unusual to specify several objectives, which, if met, suggest your goal has been achieved. In fact, you should be able to draw an arrow from each objective to your goal, indicating their connections to the ultimate purpose of the campaign.

It should be noted that your campaign may have multiple, time-oriented objectives. In other words, you may specify some short-term objectives, which, if met, lead to longer-term objectives, which, if met in turn, should lead to goal achievement. For example, an immediate, or short-term, objective might be to "increase to 90% the number of student bicyclists who can correctly identify 100% of the bicycle safety signals by the end of the first term." This initial objective in your campaign might then lead to a longer-term objective focused on cyclists' behavior, which would then lead to the goal.

Now after all objectives have been delineated, it is time to think about various activities that lead to the achievement of your objectives. Undoubtedly, numerous activities could be carried out to meet the objectives; your task is to determine, based on a number of criteria (e.g., time, budget, personnel) the best activities for your campaign. Before discussing specific activities, let's discuss a few points and an example of a comprehensive plan.

First, just as objectives should logically lead to the goal, activities should logically lead to the objectives. In other words, you should be able to draw an arrow from each activity to one or more objectives. The second, and perhaps most important, point is that activities are selected only *after* the goals and objectives have been specified. Although you may have initial ideas about activities to employ, you are further ahead in the long run if you begin with the campaign goal and work toward messages or activities, as this direction ensures the activities fit the objectives. The danger in starting with messages or activities is that a great deal of time is spent developing and planning them, but in the end, they may not lead to the fulfillment of your objectives. Of course, you may find that your initial ideas do fit one or more of the objectives and thus, you still may incorporate them into your campaign. The difference is that by following our recommendation, you begin to develop and plan the messages or activities only after you're sure they are useful in meeting your stated objectives.

A plan for a campaign focused on campus safety, and more specifically on bicycle safety, is provided in Figure 5.1. This plan began with the goal statement, "increase the bicycling safety of students at Healthy University." As discussed previously, this is a general statement reflecting the ultimate impact of the campaign. It is not directly ame-

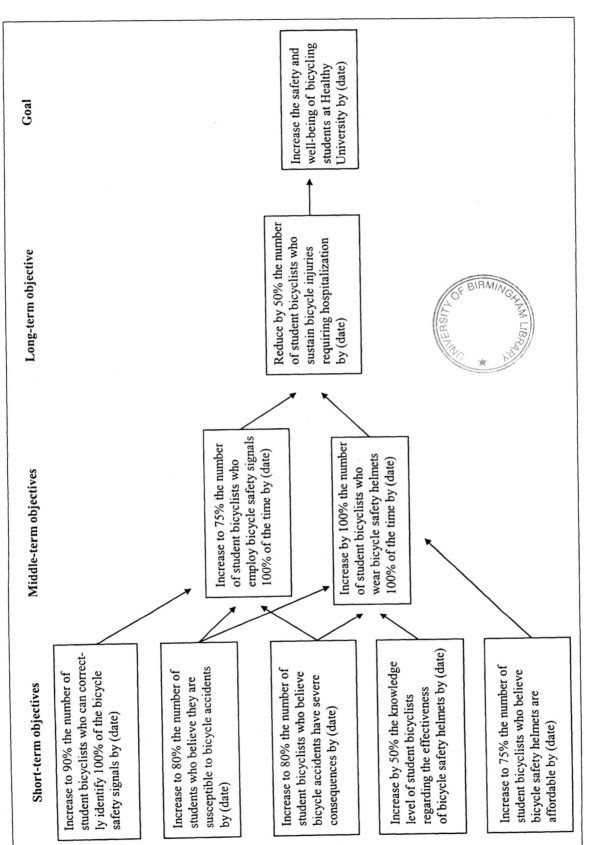

Short-term objectives

Increase to 90% the number of student bicyclists who can correctly identify 100% of the bicycle safety signals by (date)

Increase to 80% the number of students who believe they are susceptible to bicycle accidents by (date)

Increase to 80% the number of student bicyclists who believe bicycle accidents have severe consequences by (date)

Increase by 50% the knowledge level of student bicyclists regarding the effectiveness of bicycle safety helmets by (date)

Increase to 75% the number of student bicyclists who believe bicycle safety helmets are affordable by (date)

Middle-term objectives

Increase to 75% the number of student bicyclists who employ bicycle safety signals 100% of the time by (date)

Increase by 100% the number of student bicyclists who wear bicycle safety helmets 100% of the time by (date)

Long-term objective

Reduce by 50% the number of student bicyclists who sustain bicycle injuries requiring hospitalization by (date)

Goal

Increase the safety and well-being of bicycling students at Healthy University by (date)

Figure 5.1 A Campaign Plan for Setting Goals and Objectives

CHAPTER 5

nable to measurement, but fits with the university's goal of a safer campus, and thus may be measured at the "community" or university level.

The long-term objective is to "reduce by 50% the number of Healthy University students who sustain injuries requiring hospitalization from bicycle accidents by October (of specified year)." This objective statement includes an outcome (reduction by 50% of bicycle accidents requiring hospitalization), a target audience (students at Healthy U.), and a time frame (October of specified year). As such, this objective can be measured or evaluated through an outcome evaluation. An arrow is drawn from this objective to the goal signifying that fulfillment of this long-term objective should lead to the goal of a safer campus. Working back, two middle-term objectives are stated. The first middle-term objective is to "increase to 75% the number of Healthy University students who employ bicycle signals 100% of the time by May (of specified year)." Again, this objective contains an outcome, a target audience, and a time frame, which necessarily precedes the time frame for the long-term objective. The second middle-term objective is to "increase by 100% the number of Healthy University students who wear bicycle safety helmets 100% of the time by May (of specified year)." Although these two objectives differ from each other, each logically leads to the long-term objective of reducing bicycle accidents requiring hospitalization. Therefore, arrows are drawn from each of these middle-term objectives to the long-term objective.

Working back again, five short-term objectives are stated (see Figure 5.1). Each of these objectives is measurable and logically leads to one or more of the middle-term objectives. Note that two of the objectives, one focused on susceptibility and one focused on severity, have arrows leading to both of the middle-term objectives, whereas the other three short-term objectives specifically relate to only one of the middle-term objectives. This is not unusual in that the accomplishment of some objectives leads to multiple longer-term objectives, although others lead to only a single longer-term objective. Of greatest importance is that each objective leads to at least one longer-term objective, or in the case of long-term objectives, each logically leads to fulfillment of the goal.

■■ FORMATIVE RESEARCH

Now that you have developed your goals and objectives, it's time to begin your formative research. In formative research, you clearly identify your target audience, develop a prototypical member or members, and determine important demographic variables, prior experiences, beliefs, and perceptions toward your health threat and the recommended response. Formative research helps you develop targeted, culturally appropriate, health risk messages that work.

The following framework for formative research was based on a number of persuasion theories. We took the best parts of three successful and well-tested theories and combined them into a single framework (for full rationale and explication, see Witte, 1992c, 1995). Two of the main components follow the Extended Parallel Process Model.

■■ THE PERSUASIVE HEALTH MESSAGE (PHM) FRAMEWORK

For a health risk message to be effective, it must take into account the client or audience's cultural, demographic, and geographic reality. The framework described here does that

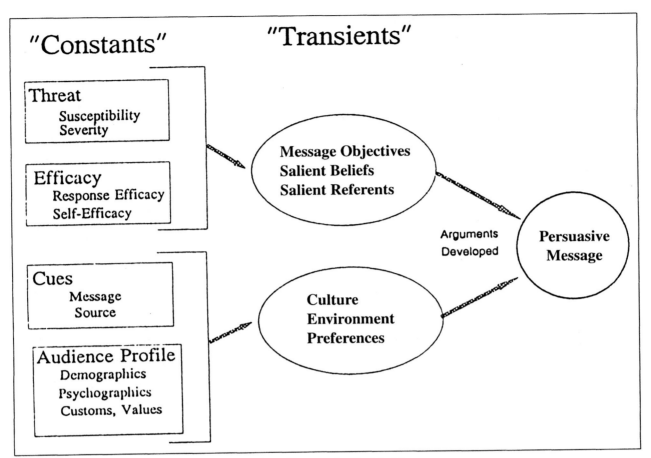

Figure 5.2 A Framework for Developing Culturally Specific Health Messages

by borrowing elements from three persuasion theories-the Theory of Reasoned Action (Fishbein & Ajzen, 1975), the Elaboration Likelihood Model (Petty & Cacioppo, 1986), and Protection Motivation Theory/Extended Parallel Process Model (Rogers, 1983; Witte, 1992a). This framework is a step-by-step approach for generating targeted and culturally-appropriate campaigns.

To begin, the PHM Framework states that you must address two separate factors when developing your health risk campaign-the "transient" and the "constant" factors (see Figure 5.2). Each of these is described in depth below. We start with the constant factors.

Health Risk Message Constants

The constant factors of a health risk message stay the same or remain the focus regardless of the health issue, no matter the composition of the target population and the type of message (e.g., interpersonal, poster, television commercial) you develop. The constant components of every health risk message are (a) the threat, (b) the efficacy of the recommended response, (c) various cues, and (d) the audience profile.

Threat and Efficacy

By now, you should be very familiar with the first two constant components, which come from Protection Motivation Theory (Rogers, 1983) and the EPPM (Witte, 1992). The threat portion of the message focuses on how susceptible the audience is to a severe threat. The efficacy portion of the message focuses on individuals' perceptions concerning their ability to perform the recommended response (i.e., self-efficacy), as well as their perceptions about how effective the recommended response is in averting the threat (i.e., response efficacy). As discussed in previous chapters, when individuals perceive high levels of threat (e.g., "I'm at risk for developing heart disease and could die from it") and high levels of efficacy (e.g., "But if I exercise daily and eat healthy, which I know I can do, I'll prevent the disease"), then they are motivated to protect themselves against the threat (Witte, 1992a, 1992b). Thus, the PHM (Persuasive Health Message) framework states that any effective health risk message should convince individuals (a) they are susceptible to a severe threat, and that (b) they are able to adopt an easy and feasible response to effectively avert the threat. Remember, people must believe they are able to perform an effective response to avert the threat, otherwise the message may backfire. Thus, the recommended response must be seen as efficacious enough to eliminate or substantially reduce the threat before people actually implement it. If people do not believe the recommended response works and/or if they don't believe they can perform it, then they focus on controlling their fear, that is, they deny or defensively avoid thinking about the health threat. In other words, they totally ignore your message and continue engaging in unhealthy behaviors (e.g., smoke more cigarettes).

Cues

The third constant component, cues, refer to those variables that can influence the persuasive process indirectly. For example, some people may not think about the content of your message or what you're actually saying, but may accept a message simply because it was delivered by a highly credible person. For example, upon hearing that your favorite sports star buys Nike tennis shoes, you may buy Nikes. You weren't persuaded to buy Nikes by arguments about the shoes' high quality or their superior construction. You simply bought Nikes because your favorite sports star did. His or her credibility/reputation/prestige convinced you Nikes must be great tennis shoes, not discussion of the quality of the leather used or the innovative construction techniques that create air pockets, and so on.

Cues tend to persuade via the peripheral route, according to the Elaboration Likelihood Model. If you recall, the Elaboration Likelihood Model suggests when people are persuaded via the peripheral route, they are not thinking about or evaluating the content of the message; instead, they are using mental models such as "he's an expert; if he does it then I'll do it" or "if my favorite celebrity does X then I will, too." Cues are anything that prompts decision making without consideration of the message. For example, attractiveness, similarity in source (e.g., "she comes from the same neighborhood as I do so if she's doing it then I should, too."), trustworthiness (e.g., a respected person in your community), expertise (e.g., a doctor, dentist, optometrist, says to do it, so it must be OK), number of arguments (lots of arguments must be better than just one), can all act as peripheral cues that cause you to adopt a recommended response without thinking about the message. When people do not have the ability and/or motivation to process a message centrally (i.e., they don't have the ability and/or motivation to think about the message content), then they process it peripherally (as long as a peripheral cue is present).

At least two variables typically act as cues in health risk messages-source and message type. Source variables are related to the source of a message, such as credibility, attractiveness, similarity to receiver, power, and so on (McGuire, 1984). Message variables refer to non-content issues such as organization of the message (e.g., threat first, then efficacy, OR efficacy first, then threat), type of appeal (e.g., humorous, logical, emotional), number of repetitions in a message, vividness of language, and so on (McGuire, 1984). Although these variables act as cues when a message is processed peripherally, source and message variables also can act as arguments and be carefully considered in a central route-processing manner. For example, in a shampoo commercial, you may carefully think about the consistency and texture of a model's beautiful hair, and you may carefully evaluate whether the shampoo really led to thicker, more vibrant, and bouncy hair. More likely, however, you just use the model's hair as a peripheral cue, that is, "her hair looks good, so if I use the shampoo mine will too."

Cues are important to address in health risk messages because even though you may prefer your audience centrally processes the message, at least some audience members are not motivated or able to do so. Therefore, you need to include persuasive cues in your health risk message to persuade your entire audience-those who are motivated and able as well as those who are unmotivated or unable to process your messages.

Audience Profile

The final constant component is the audience profile. Developing an audience profile prior to your campaign is important because it helps you tailor your message to your specific audience. If your target audience is composed of two or three distinct groups of people with some commonalties, you may wish to develop two or three audience profiles with the common links specified. At a minimum, gather demographics (e.g., age, sex, occupation, education, native language), psychographics (e.g., lifestyle practices), and information on cultural beliefs and values (e.g., role of the family, relation between religion and health).

Having this information helps develop a targeted health risk message from the audience's point-of-view instead of your own. Developing a message according to the audience's point-of-view is critical. In our research, we have often found that our target audience or clients have totally different ways of viewing the world than we do-sometimes in ways unfathomable to us. For example, in one study on HIV/AIDS prevention in Kenya, we had a difficult time understanding a point commercial sex workers were making about the inadequacy of condoms. As you may know, when you purchase condoms, they often come in packs of three. The commercial sex workers kept saying that they'd use the condoms initially but then as the night wore on, they'd go "steel-to-steel" (i.e., skin-to-skin). We couldn't understand why the condoms wouldn't work during sexual intercourse. Eventually, it came out that it was normal to have sex five to seven times a night with the same client and that a package of three condoms simply wasn't enough for even a single night's work! We did not even consider the possibility that the reason condoms weren't working for the commercial sex workers was because there simply weren't enough of them in a package for an evening's work. We were trapped in our worldview of American culture where it is normative to have sex once or maybe twice a night. Without formative research, we would have developed messages that promoted condoms, showed the correct way to use them, and made them available (in our limited perception) to commercial sex workers. However, our notions of availability (i.e., one or two condoms a night) differed significantly from what an adequate supply of condoms really was for the Kenyan commercial sex workers. Condoms distributed in packs of three are perfectly fine for an American audience, but grossly inadequate for a Kenyan audience. It is important to keep an open mind when forming an audience analysis and go beyond what you define as possible based on your background and experience. It is dangerous to assume that all audiences and/or clients live their lives or perceive their world as we do.

Health Risk Message Transients

Health risk message transients are the parts of a message that shift depending on the target population and health issue. The transients parts of a message are changeable elements (recall the constants stay the same). The transient information gathered in formative research fills in the constant components of the message. The transient information includes beliefs, cultural background, demographics, and everything that determines the actual features and content of a message.

Two categories of transient information need to be specified. First, the objectives of your health risk message must be clearly and explicitly stated in relation to your health threat and the recommended response. What is the exact health issue of concern? What are the specific responses recommended to avert or decrease the threat? The more specific your objectives, the better your message is and the greater influence it has on your audience. For example, your health threat may be HIV/AIDS infection and your recommended response may be to use condoms. Although these are fairly specific, they can be made even more explicit. Do you want people to use condoms all of the time, only with one-night stands, or only with their regular partners? A more specific recommended response is "use condoms each time you have sex." Then, you need to determine salient beliefs about the threat and efficacy of the recommended response.

Salient beliefs are the first five to seven responses elicited when your audience is asked a question. For example, if asked, "what do you like about this class," your first five to seven responses are your salient beliefs about this class. In addition to salient beliefs, salient referents and beliefs about salient referents' perceptions need to be ascertained (recall the discussion on the theory of reasoned action).

Salient referents are people who have an influence on your opinion of the recommended response. Your parents may be salient referents about immunizations (i.e., they strongly influence your beliefs about immunization). Your sexual partner may be your salient referent for using condoms or birth control. Research has shown that subjective norms, or what you think your salient referents think and whether you are motivated to comply with them, have a large influence on behavior (see Theory of Reasoned Action in Chapter 4). Subjective norms are explained further below.

The second category of transient information to be gathered is culture/environment information and preferences. This information is used to develop cues and the audience profile. To begin, find out from whom your target audience wants to hear about the health risk-a doctor, a celebrity, someone similar to themselves? Then, determine what type of message the audience prefers-an emotional appeal or logical information? Next, determine which channel the audience prefers-radio, TV, or newspaper? Finally, develop an audience profile from the cultural (e.g., demographics, psychographics) and environmental information (e.g., characteristics of the audience's immediate environment, accessibility and/or availability of transportation to services/products) you've gathered.

An audience analysis enables you to gather the transient information to provide details for the constant components. The format for the audience analysis is based on Fishbein and Ajzen's (1975, 1981) Theory of Reasoned Action. Fishbein and Ajzen (1975) argue that to change a behavior, you must change the underlying set of salient beliefs causing a specific behavior. For instance, if the specific behavior is wearing seatbelts, and you believe "seatbelts are uncomfortable; seatbelts trap you if you go under water; seatbelts protect against rear end collisions," and "seatbelts trap you if your car catches on fire," then changing only a single belief about seatbelts is unlikely to influence your overall behavior because the other remaining beliefs keep you from wearing seatbelts. In addition, the Theory of Reasoned Action suggests that you need to find out the audience's subjective norm with reference to the recommended behavior. The subjective norm is comprised of (a) what individuals believe salient referents think about the performance of behavior X, and (b) the individual's motivation to comply with the salient referent (see Chapter 4; Fishbein & Ajzen, 1975). In other words, your target audience's salient beliefs about a health threat, salient referents (e.g., best friend, significant other, parents), beliefs about their salient referents (e.g., my best friend/significant other/parents think I should. . .), and motivation to comply with the beliefs of their salient referents (e.g., I am [not] highly motivated to do what my best friend/significant other/parents think I should do) all affect the audience's subjective norm related to the threat. For example, to increase the wearing of seatbelts, it is necessary to find out the audience's important referents in terms of seatbelt wearing and what your audience believes is their referents' opinions about their wearing seatbelts. Finally, you need to find out whether the audience is motivated to comply with those referents. For instance, say that friends, lovers, and parents are salient referents to your target audience. Most of your audience believes that parents want them to wear seatbelts but friends and lovers don't because they're too constricting. The audience is more motivated to comply with friends and lovers than with parents, so for the most part, they do not wear the seatbelt as a result of this negative subjective norm.

Overall, according to the Theory of Reasoned Action, to truly change behavior you must (a) uncover the whole set of salient beliefs toward the advocated behavior, both good and bad, and (b) develop a message that refutes beliefs that inhibit the behavior and promotes beliefs that encourage the behavior. Once the transient information (i.e., salient beliefs and referents) for each of the constant components is determined, then the messages can be developed.

PUTTING TRANSIENTS AND CONSTANTS TOGETHER ▪▪

Once you've gathered the transient information, then you simply plug it into the constant components of the framework and develop your message. The use of transient information to inform the constant components of a message works for several reasons. First, focusing on the audience's specific salient beliefs about the threat and efficacy of the recommended response increases involvement in and the personal relevancy of the message. Not only does focusing on salient beliefs increase the audience's motivation to process a message, it also makes the message more understandable because it addresses their specific issues. Thus, their ability to process the message is increased as well. Remember, increased motivation and ability to process a message causes the message to be centrally processed, which leads to lasting and stable behavior change (Petty & Cacioppo, 1986). However, sometimes your audience is too tired or preoccupied to process the message centrally, no matter how relevant and easy it is to understand. This is why cues must be included in your health risk message. The audience analysis should have provided insights about preferred message sources, cultural issues, demographic issues, and so on. Be sure to include as many culturally acceptable cues as possible in your message. By doing this, you may peripherally persuade those who are unmotivated or unable to process your message centrally. Using the PHM approach increases your chances of persuading an audience through the central route, as well as enabling you to affect audience members who don't care or aren't interested in the message via the peripheral route.

Now you have the theoretical background to engage in formative research. In the following section are step-by-step procedures for conducting a formative evaluation with the PHM framework.

■ GATHERING INFORMATION FOR THE PERSUASIVE HEALTH MESSAGE FRAMEWORK

Three simple steps lead to the development of risk messages through the PHM framework. Several worksheets are provided in the worksheets section to help you develop your messages.

Step 1: Determine Goals and Objectives of the Health Risk Message: Questions to Ask Yourself

First, you need to carefully define the parameters of the constant components. As such, provide the most specific response possible to the following questions when beginning to design your health risk message (see Worksheet 10, Questions for the Health Risk Message Developer).

1. What is the threat you are trying to prevent?

2. What is the recommended response to avert the threat (the *specific* objective of the campaign)?

3. Who is the target audience (be specific)?

Question 1 is important because an awareness of a threat tends to *motivate* individuals to act. Although it may not be immediately apparent, nearly all health risk messages try to prevent some type of threat from occurring. For example, if you're promoting exercise, a seemingly positive behavior with no negative consequences, then you're ultimately trying to prevent cancer or heart disease. Remember, perceived threats and their associated negative consequences should ultimately be determined by your target audience because they may perceive threats and negative consequences very differently than you do. Nonetheless, this worksheet will get you started with some general ideas.

Question 2 should represent the specific objective of your campaign and should be as quantifiable as possible. For example, "improving daily nutrition" is a measurable objective, but "increasing (a) the number of vegetables eaten each day and (b) the number of fruits eaten each day" is a better, more specific objective. In any health risk message, the recommended response is the immediate objective or focus of the campaign (e.g., condom use) with the belief that the ultimate goal (e.g., HIV/AIDS prevention) can be achieved through adoption of this recommended response (i.e., prevent HIV/AIDS infection by advocating condom use).

Question 3 allows you to develop a profile of the audience so the message can be targeted toward this specific audience. Be sure to define the target population according to demographic varianles (e.g., beliefs, values, worldview), and culture (e.g., customs, norms). Answers to question 3 are especially important in any risk message targeted toward a group different than yourself (i.e., a different ethnic group, a different social group, etc.).

Step 2:   Ask Audience Members Questions to Determine Salient Beliefs, Recommended Responses, Salient Referents, Source/Channel Preferences, and Stage of Readiness

The second step is to survey a small sample of your target audience (as you've defined in #3 above) to find out their salient beliefs, referents, and preferences. Four worksheets are included in this step (Worksheets 11, 12, 13, and 14). Each of these can be administered separately or at the same time to your sample from your target audience. How many people you survey is really up to you, but we recommend that you survey at least 10 people. Chapter 9 provides additional detail concerning the methods for drawing an appropriate sample. Even if you can't follow these scientific principles, surveying several people who fit your audience profile will increase the appropriateness and effectiveness of your message tremendously. As an aside, we have found that focus groups (discussion sessions with six to nine individuals in a group setting) are *not* good methodological tools to gather salient beliefs because people's perceptions may be colored by what other members of the group say. You won't get "pure" unbiased perceptions about a health threat or recommended response if you ask a whole group what it thinks. It's best to have members of the target audience answer these questions individually, for example, in an interview. When it's time to get feedback on campaign messages or materials, then focus groups work well. We have found, however, that they don't work when you're trying to gather salient beliefs and perceptions. Therefore, it is preferable to ask these questions of individuals in face-to-face interviews.

To determine salient beliefs, referents, preferences, and cultural beliefs, you can either survey a small sample of your target audience or you can review existing research. First, ask open-ended questions to find out your audience's honest and untainted perceptions about the threat and recommended response. Second, find out salient referents by determining which individuals or groups have the most influence on targeted audience members with reference to the specified threat and the recommended response. If you use existing research, answer the questions with what ethnographers or others have *found*. Here are some examples of questions designed to elicit salient beliefs (see also Worksheet 11).

1. What are your beliefs about [PERFORMING THE RECOMMENDED RESPONSE]? *(this is your attitude toward recommended response)*

2. What negative consequences, if any, come from not [PERFORMING RECOMMENDED RESPONSE]? *determines audience perceptions of the threat)*

3. What is the best way to prevent experiencing the negative consequences just identified? *(determines audience perceptions of the "best" recommended response)*

4. Please list the people or groups who have an important influence on your [USING THE RECOMMENDED RESPONSE]? *(referents for subjective norm)*

Once you've determined what members of your audience find threatening and what motivates them to perform the recommended health behavior, then you'll want to determine specific salient beliefs about the threat, the efficacy of the recommended response, and beliefs about what the audience members think salient referents think about the threat and recommended response. The following questions also ascertain salient beliefs about barriers and benefits to performing the recommended response. According to the Health Belief Model (Chapter 4), these variables, especially barriers, are important contributors to health behaviors. See also Worksheet 12.

1. How serious is [THREAT/NEGATIVE CONSEQUENCES]? Please explain. *(perceived severity of the threat)*

2. How likely is it that you will experience the [THREAT/NEGATIVE CONSEQUENCES] if you do not [PERFORMING THE RECOMMENDED RESPONSE]? Please explain. *(perceived susceptibility of the threat)*

3. Do you believe the {RECOMMENDED RESPONSE] will prevent you from experiencing the [THREAT/NEGATIVE CONSEQUENCES]? Why or why not? *(perceived response efficacy)*

4. Do you believe you are easily able to perform the [RECOMMENDED RESPONSE] to prevent you from experiencing the [THREAT/NEGATIVE CONSEQUENCES]? Why or why not? *(perceived self-efficacy)*

5. What might keep you from performing the [RECOMMENDED RESPONSE]? Please explain. *(perceived benefits)*

6. What benefits do you perceive from performing the {RECOMMENDED RESPONSE]? Please explain. *(perceived benefit)*

It is very important to ask open-ended questions such as these of members of your target audience because even though you feel you know your audience and how they'll answer, you may be surprised (and probably will be). For example, everyone knows that to promote birth control, the biggest threat you can use to motivate action is to say you'll get pregnant and have a baby if you don't. Right? Wrong. Remember the study we described in Chapter 1? If you recall, we described a formative evaluation we did of inner-city teens where the researchers had defined the "threat" from not using birth control as "getting pregnant and having a baby." However, we found that most of these inner-city teens did not view having a baby as a negative consequence; in fact, they viewed it as a benefit. The real threat of pregnancy was "getting fat"-a terrible threat that was greatly feared by these appearance-conscious teenagers. Thus, this study showed us that the best threat to use to motivate adoption of the recommended response (i.e., birth control) was the threat of "getting fat" from being pregnant. This study shows us it is critical to find out what the *audience* perceives the negative consequences are from not performing the recommended response, not what you think they are.

In addition to open-ended questions similar like these, it is sometimes useful to use a closed-ended questionnaire to determine levels of perceived threat and efficacy toward the recommended responses. Open-ended questions let respondents answer without setting parameters, while closed-ended questions give several responses and ask respondents to choose just one. Open-ended questions are needed because you need to gather "pure" salient beliefs without imposing your beliefs on the audience. Closed-ended questions, however, may be needed to determine whether audiences feel susceptible to the threat, feel the threat is severe, believe they can perform the recommended response, and believe the recommended response works in averting the threat. Some examples of closed-ended questions follow (see also Worksheet 13).

1. I am at-risk for [EXPERIENCING THE THREAT]. *(perceived susceptibility)*

1	2	3	4	5	6	7
Strongly Disagree						Strongly Agree

2. [THE THREAT] is serious. *(perceived severity)*

1	2	3	4	5	6	7
Strongly Disagree						Strongly Agree

3. [PERFORMING THE RECOMMENDED RESPONSE] will prevent [THE THREAT]. *(perceived response efficacy)*

1	2	3	4	5	6	7
Strongly Disagree						Strongly Agree

4. I am easily able to [PERFORM THE RECOMMENDED RESPONSE]. *(perceived self-efficacy)*

1	2	3	4	5	6	7
Strongly Disagree						Strongly Agree

Finally, it's time to gather information for your cues and audience profile. Demographic information available from census records and data from survey research can be used to create a profile. The following preference information can be gathered directly from a sample of your target audience. In addition, we have developed questions to determine which stage of readiness your audience is in, based on the Stages of Change Model (see Chapter 4). Feel free to add questions related to cultural values, medical practices, health-related customs, and so on, to enhance the profile. Here are some examples of items to use to gather audience information (see also Worksheet 14).

1. Please rank order the ways in which you prefer to learn about the [RECOM-MENDED RESPONSE], with "1" representing your most preferred way of learning about the recommended response and "7" representing your least preferred way of learning about the recommended response. *(preferred channel)*

    _____ television

    _____ magazine

    _____ newspaper

    _____ internet

    _____ radio

    _____ interpersonal (face-to-face) channel

    _____ other (specify) _____

2. Please rank order who would you believe most to who you would believe least regarding a message on the [RECOMMENDED RESPONSE], with "1" representing who you'd believe most and "7" representing who you'd believe least? *(preferred source)*

    _____ health care professional

    _____ celebrity

    _____ Surgeon General

    _____ my parents

    _____ my colleagues

    _____ my friends

    _____ other (specify) _____

3. Please rank order the type of message you'd like to receive most for this [RECOM-MENDED RESPONSE], with "1" representing your most preferred message type and "7" representing your least preferred message type.

    _____ message with lots of facts

    _____ entertaining message

    _____ comic-type message

    _____ message using stories of real people's experiences

    _____ message with good arguments

    _____ message that influences me emotionally

    _____ scary message

    _____ other type of message: _____

4. Respond "yes" or "no" to each of the following statements concerning your thoughts and actions. *(stage of change)*

    a. _____ Yes _____ No

       I have thought about [DOING RECOMMENDED RESPONSE]. *(precontemplation)*

    b. _____ Yes _____ No

       I have thought about [DOING RECOMMENDED RESPONSE] but have not taken any steps to [DO IT] yet. *(contemplation)*

    c. _____ Yes _____ No

       I have not yet [DONE RECOMMENDED RESPONSE] but have taken steps so that I will be able to soon (e.g., GIVE EXAMPLES). *(preparation—never used)*

d. _____ Yes _____ No
    I have [DONE RECOMMENDED RESPONSE]. *(action)*

e. _____ Yes _____ No
    I regularly [DO RECOMMENDED RESPONSE]. *(maintenance)*

f. _____ Yes _____ No
    I have [DONE RECOMMENDED RESPONSE] before but currently do
    not [DO IT]. *(relapse . . . go to either preparation or contemplation stage)*

Step 3 Developing Your Health Risk Message

At this step, you are ready to develop the message. You have already defined your goals and objectives (Step 1) and conducted your audience research (Step 2). Now you will analyze the data gathered in Step 2 in line with your stated goals and objectives (Step 1) and develop your messages based on this analysis. There are four things you need to do in Step 3 to develop your message:

a. Develop one or more prototypical members of your audience (maximum three) based on your audience analysis information gathered in Step 1, question #3. These prototypical characters you create should be used in any health risk messages. The characters represent the individuals experiencing the health threat.

b. List source, channel, and message preferences for your audience based on information gathered in Step 2. For any final message, you should use the preferred source, channel, and message type indicated by your audience analysis. For example, if the majority of your audience prefers fear-arousing messages delivered by a celebrity over the radio, then your final message should be delivered by a celebrity in a radio announcement and the message should arouse fear in some manner.

c. Identify which stage of change your target audience is in from the last question asked in Step 2 (e.g., precontemplation, contemplation, preparation, action, maintenance). Knowing the stage of change of your audience enables you to develop messages that move them from one stage to the next. For example, if your audience is completely unaware of the health threat (precontemplation stage), your messages will need to create awareness and knowledge about the health threat. Or, if your audience is already performing the behavior (action or maintenance stage), then your messages will need to reinforce current behavioral patterns. Refer to the discussion in Chapter 4 on what types of messages to use given a certain Stage of Change if you're not quite sure what to do regarding moving people from one stage to the next.

d. Next, develop a chart to categorize responses to Worksheets 11, 12, and 13. This chart facilitates the development of your health risk messages because it identifies your audience's important beliefs and tells you whether you should reinforce, refute, or introduce new beliefs. The chart is described in more detail in the next section.

e. Now you can develop your message. Simply use your prototypical audience member as the character(s) in your message. Utilize the preferred channels, sources, and message types. Use message appeals that address the appropriate stage of change (e.g., knowledge messages, motivational messages, etc.). Finally, develop specific arguments that either refute, reinforce, or introduce beliefs according to your chart, which was based on your audience research in Worksheets 11, 12, and 13 (described next). Your final product should be an effective, targeted, and theoretically based message that is culturally appropriate for your audience.

⊞ CATEGORIZING AUDIENCE BELIEFS: A CHART TO GUIDE MESSAGE DEVELOPMENT

Step 2 questions gathered salient beliefs and referents regarding the health threat and the recommended response. Now, these beliefs need to be organized and categorized so they can be addressed in the health risk message. Overall, at least three types of arguments can be made in a persuasive message. A message can try to change beliefs, reinforce existing beliefs, or introduce new beliefs (Burgoon, 1989; McGuire, 1985). It is much easier to reinforce and strengthen existing beliefs or introduce new beliefs in a health risk message than it is to try to change existing and entrenched beliefs (Rice & Atkin, 2001). The most effective health risk message is compatible with the target audience's existing beliefs, attitudes, and behaviors (Rogers, 1995). In this type of message, little counter-argument and defensiveness result because the message reinforces and supports your audience's existing belief structure. Thus, it is helpful to frame the recommended response as fitting within the target audience's current belief and value system.

As a hypothetical example, let us presume that members of a certain cultural group do not care about their health, but family is of utmost importance to them. Then, the recommended response should be framed so it leads to the protection and promotion of the family (e.g., "Who will take care of them? If you stay healthy, you can!"). In summary, the responses to Step 2's questions on Worksheets 11 and 12 should be put into one of three categories:

- Beliefs to refute or change
- Beliefs to reinforce or strengthen
- Beliefs to introduce

But, how do you know which beliefs to reinforce, to refute (change), and to introduce? The theory you choose to guide your project tells you the beliefs that need addressing in a message and the direction these messages should take (i.e., positive or negative). For example, we know from the EPPM that perceptions of susceptibility, severity, response efficacy, and self-efficacy should all be at high levels for the most effective message. We also know that perceptions of response and self-efficacy must be stronger than perceptions of susceptibility and severity, or we risk developing a message that backfires and leads to fear control responses such as denial or reactance. We also know from descriptions of other theories that perceived barriers need to be minimized (minimizing barriers also increases perceived efficacy; i.e., if a person does not feel able to perform the recommended response because of barriers, then the removal of those barriers increases their perceived ability to perform the recommended response).

Therefore, we've identified five beliefs to be addressed in a message-susceptibility, severity, response efficacy, self-efficacy, and barriers. We've also addressed the direction these beliefs should go. Response efficacy and self-efficacy should be very strong and

Table 5.1   Grateful Med Belief Chart

Audience Profile	Beliefs to Change	Beliefs to Reinforce	Beliefs to Introduce
High literacy level; over age 50	Grateful Med is hard to use	I need up-to-date info to effectively treat my patients	Grateful Med has new services that help me search quickly and efficiently for info
Tend to be computer illiterate; use typewriters	It takes too long to find the info I need on Grateful Med	Grateful Med contains the info I need	
Extremely stressed, overwhelmed by daily commitments	I don't have enough time to use Grateful Med	. . . (fill in more)	Within 10 minutes you can be up and running on Grateful Med because of a new, easy-to-use tutorial
Live in rural area; few colleagues use Internet	. . . (fill in more)		. . . (fill in more)
. . . (fill in more)			

positive; susceptibility and severity also should be strong but not so strong that they lead to feelings of powerlessness in the face of the threat. Barriers should be reduced or eliminated. If the audience research indicates no salient beliefs emerged for any of these five beliefs, then the message should introduce these beliefs in the desired direction (e.g., promote strong perceptions of susceptibility, decrease perceptions of barriers, etc.).

A belief chart we developed to promote Grateful Med, an Internet service that specializes in medical information, is reproduced in Table 5.1. Our target audience was rural medical practitioners, such as doctors and nurses. We defined the threat as "being out of date regarding medical practices, which can potentially result in harm to patients." The recommended response was "use Grateful Med frequently to keep up-to-date on current medical knowledge." Most of our target audience was in the precontemplation or contemplation stage, so messages focused on increasing their awareness of Grateful Med and motivation to use it. Audience members' responses to the questions listed in Step 2 and in Worksheets 11 and 12 were placed into Table 5.1.

Address each belief listed in Table 5.1 according to whether it should be reinforced, refuted, or introduced. To maximize effectiveness, the arguments in your health risk message should directly address the audience's salient beliefs. Ideally, each salient belief gathered in your formative research should be reinforced (ideally) or refuted (if necessary) in the health risk message. However, if the health risk message is limited by space or time, only the most salient beliefs may be targeted (i.e., only those beliefs listed by all members of your audience). Also, if time is a factor, use the closed-ended items found in Step 2. These items indicate whether the audience believes the threat is severe, whether they believe they are susceptible to the threat, whether they believe the recommended response works, and whether they believe they can perform the recommended response. You can place their responses to these closed-ended questions into categories to change, reinforce, or introduce, as well. For example, if the audience strongly disagrees that they are susceptible to the threat, you know you need to change that belief so they feel susceptible to the threat. If your audience members mark "4" for the response efficacy and self-efficacy questions, indicating a neutral response, then you may need to introduce beliefs about the ease and effectiveness of the recommended response.

Now you know all the steps for developing an effective, culturally appropriate health risk message. To summarize,

1. Determine goals and objectives of the health risk message (Step 1 and Worksheet 10).

2. Conduct formative research by either face-to-face or telephone interviews, typically using paper-and-pencil surveys (Step 2 and Worksheets 11, 12, 13, 14).

3. Develop an audience profile by writing a complete description of the "typical" member of your target audience; include lifestyle practices, cultural beliefs, religious values, and so on (Step 2 or Worksheet 11, question 3).

4. List source, channel, and message preferences and salient referents; visual or audio elements of the message (non-content aspects of the message) should fit the target audience's cultural values, demographic characteristics, specific needs, and source/channel preferences (Step 2 or Worksheet 14, question 4).

5. Determine stage of change readiness for most of your audience and list ideas for moving them into the next stage (Step 2 or Worksheet 14, question 3).

6. Categorize salient beliefs into a chart of beliefs to change, reinforce, or introduce (Step 2 or Worksheets 11, 12, 13; see chart development under Step 3).

7. Use theory to guide development of the message (see Step 3).

   Develop persuasive arguments that make the audience feel susceptible to a significant and serious threat. Check beliefs chart to see if audience already perceives threat in this manner. Develop messages to change, reinforce, or introduce beliefs.

   Develop persuasive arguments that make the audience believe the recommended response effectively, easily, and feasibly averts the threat. This section should make the audience believe they can easily perform the recommended response. Any perceived barriers should be fully addressed and refuted (e.g., if transportation is a problem, provide information about public transportation to health clinics; if cost is a problem, identify free clinics or low-cost alternatives).

8. Keeping all this in mind, be creative and have fun.

9. Evaluate and refine your message (see Chapter 9); obtain feedback on your initial drafts of the health risk messages in focus groups to make sure they produce the response desired; make sure beliefs are in the proper direction according to your theory (e.g., high threat/high efficacy messages if the EPPM is used); modify as needed; repeat pilot evaluation if necessary.

⫶ CONCLUSION

This chapter outlines one way to conduct a complete formative evaluation. As stated earlier, we believe that up-front work saves tail-end work. We believe that health risk messages developed in the manner described in this chapter are strong and effective. In the next chapter, we describe some shortcuts to developing effective health risk messages.

6

The Risk Behavior
Diagnosis Scale

Chapter 5 provided a thorough technique for conducting formative research to develop effective health risk messages. But what happens if you're out in the field and you need to rapidly develop an effective health risk message based on answers to only a few questions? Or say you're an HIV counselor or tester, or a nutritionist, or a physician, and you want to develop an effective message for each of your clients or patients on the spot. What do you do?

The Risk Behavior Diagnosis Scale (Witte, Cameron, McKeon, & Berkowitz, 1996) was developed for just these reasons. It is a rapid assessment tool that allows practitioners to quickly identify where their audience is in terms of salient beliefs about the threat and the efficacy of the recommended response and offers guidelines for developing effective health risk messages.

The Risk Behavior Diagnosis Scale—or the RBD Scale—is a 12-item survey theoretically grounded in the EPPM. Briefly, the scale asks three questions each about perceptions of severity, susceptibility, response efficacy, and self-efficacy. A quick quantitative analysis of the answers identifies whether a client/patient/audience is in fear control or danger control. You then develop your targeted health risk message on the basis of this information.

THE ORIGIN OF THE RBD SCALE ▪▪

A consistent issue of concern in the health communication field is the lack of interaction between researchers and practitioners. We researchers conduct careful experiments and surveys to determine what works and then sit back and expect practitioners to pick up where we left off. The problem is that our articles are often full of jargon and statistical mumbo-jumbo and are rarely user-friendly. At the same time, practitioners rarely have enough time to read extremely narrowly focused research articles that dissect one small component of a major theory. To solve this problem, one of the authors and her research team collaborated with the campus health center at Michigan State University with the goal of taking the EPPM and turning it into something usable by health practitioners in the field. The result was the Risk Behavior Diagnosis Scale. In this chapter, we describe the rationale and mechanics of using the scale. Chapter 7 describes real-life examples of how the scale has been used at our campus health center.

▪▪ THEORETICAL BASIS FOR EXPANDING THE EPPM

We learned in Chapter 3 that according to the EPPM, a health risk can induce one of three responses in individuals: (a) no response, (b) fear control response, or (c) danger control response. No response means that people ignored your health risk message. A fear control response means your audience rejected your message and may have done the opposite of what the message recommended, such as smoke more cigarettes. A danger control response means your audience made the recommended healthy behavior changes. Our goal then is to always induce danger control processes and responses with our health risk messages. Specifically, we want people to have strong perceptions of threat and efficacy so they are motivated to think about the health threat and adopt recommended responses.

According to the EPPM, a health risk message induces perceptions of threat and efficacy, which combine to produce either no response or the danger control or fear control processes. Therefore, if we can determine people's perceptions of threat and efficacy toward a health threat and recommended response, then we can predict which of the three responses they will engage in. Finding out someone's threat and efficacy perceptions also lets us know which perceptions need to be increased and/or decreased to promote danger control responses. Again, our goal is to always promote strong perceptions of threat (i.e., susceptibility and severity) to motivate action, and even stronger perceptions of efficacy (i.e., response efficacy and self-efficacy) to motivate the right kind of action (i.e., danger control responses such as healthy behaviors). The following EPPM concepts are important to our understanding of the RBD Scale.

The Critical Point

A key concept in the EPPM, the critical point, occurs when perceptions of threat begin to outweigh perceptions of efficacy, causing people to shift from danger control to fear control processes. Thus, the point at which individuals begin to believe they cannot effectively avert a significant and relevant threat from occurring is the critical point. This point occurs when individuals give up controlling the danger and turn instead to controlling their fear. When individuals focus on controlling their fear through responses such as denial, defensive avoidance, or reactance, they are not protecting themselves against health threats. For example, previous research has shown that fear control processes interfere with danger control processes, such that the stronger the fear control responses are, the weaker the danger control responses. In other words, if you are defensively avoiding any thoughts about a health threat, you are not making the behavioral changes necessary to protect yourself. For example, Figure 6.1-A shows an example of when the critical point occurs immediately, yielding only danger control or fear control responses. Thus, as perceptions of threat increase, either the message's recommendations are accepted (danger control) or rejected (fear control), dependent on one's level of perceived efficacy. These circumstances might occur when people have

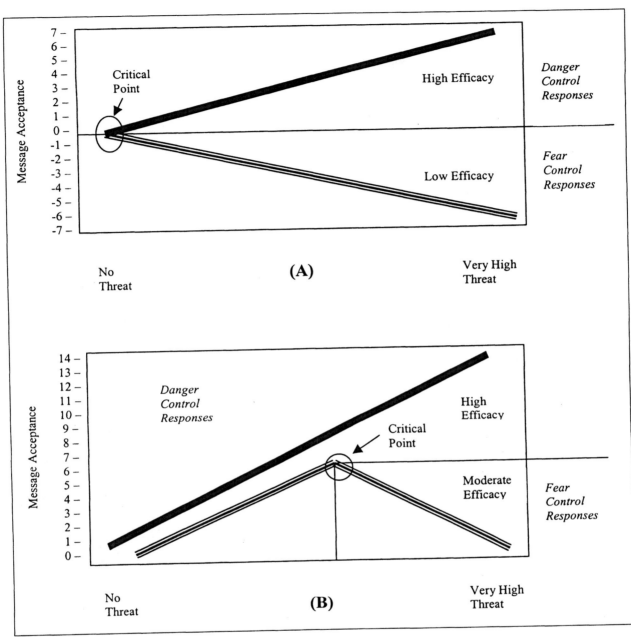

Figure 6.1 The Interaction of Threat and Efficacy

preexisting perceptions of efficacy that are either weak or strong. For example, one group might believe it can do something to avert a threat like meningitis, while another group might believe there's nothing it can do to avert meningitis. It there is no imminent meningitis threat in the area, there is no response to the threat (hence, "0" levels of message acceptance under "no threat"). But, if all of a sudden there is a meningitis outbreak, you might see a split as is shown in Figure 6.1-A, such that as people feel more and more threatened, there is more and more action—both positive and negative action. For those with high efficacy perceptions, the message's recommendations are accepted and followed as perceptions of threat increase (a danger control response). For those with low efficacy perceptions, defensive avoidance, denial, or reactance increase and the message is rejected when perceptions of threat increase (fear control responses).

In contrast, Figure 6.1-B shows a different placement of the critical value. In this example, perceived efficacy is either at a high or moderate level. As perceived threat increases in this example, people engage in danger control actions and begin to carry out a message's recommendations. At some point, however, the threat becomes too great and individuals begin to doubt their self-efficacy or the efficacy of the recommended response. At this point, they begin to ignore the message's recommendations and instead focus on controlling their fear. The purpose of the RBD scale is for you to diagnose where your audience is in their perceptions of threat and efficacy, in order to circumvent or diminish any fear control responses.

Figure 6.1 demonstrates how threat and efficacy interact to produce a critical point. The RBD Scale allows you to place a numerical value on the critical point via a simple mathematical formula. This numerical value is a hypothetical value that offers a rough distinction between those in fear control and those in danger control. The exact value of the critical point varies across different health topics and individuals. We call this simple mathematical formula the "discriminating value" formula because it discriminates between those in fear control and those in danger control.

■■ THE RBD SCALE

The RBD Scale is a 12-item scale that assesses your client's or audience's perceptions of response efficacy, self-efficacy, severity, and susceptibility on a 7-point scale ranging from "1—strongly disagree" to "7—strongly agree." Table 6.1 is a template for the RBD Scale. You simply fill in your specific health threat and your recommended response to tailor the scale to your needs.

The template for this scale (Table 6.1) has been used for many different health topics and populations and has yielded reliable and valid responses, meaning it consistently measures what it is supposed to measure. Please note that there are many variations of the RBD Scale. You choose the wording of your items to best represent your threat and recommended response. If an item doesn't seem to be working as written—for example, everyone is responding to it the same way even though you know they should differ on it—modify it until some variation in response occurs so you know it's working.

Clients respond to your version of the RBD Scale by circling numbers 1 through 7 for each item. Some very simple mathematical calculations (addition and subtraction) lead to a "discriminating score" that tells whether your audience is in fear control or danger control. Once you know this, you can develop effective health risk messages that produce high levels of danger control actions, meaning you can develop messages that result in the necessary behavioral changes. Following is a step-by-step description of how to use the RBD Scale.

Using the Scale

The steps to using the RBD Scale are simple and easy. First, clearly define your specific health threat and recommended response. Second, adopt or develop your own version of the RBD Scale using the template in Table 6.1. Third, administer the RBD Scale to your client or a sample of the target audience. Fourth, add the numerical scores for the perceived efficacy items together and add the numerical scores for the perceived

Table 6.1   A Template for the Risk Behavior Diagnosis Scale

Response Efficacy

---

1. [Performing Recommended Response] prevents [Health Threat].

1	2	3	4	5	6	7
Strongly Disagree						Strongly Agree

2. [Performing Recommended Response] works in deterring [Health Threat].

1	2	3	4	5	6	7
Strongly Disagree						Strongly Agree

3. [Performing Recommended Response] is effective in getting rid of [Health Threat].

1	2	3	4	5	6	7
Strongly Disagree						Strongly Agree

Self-Efficacy

---

4. I am able to [Perform Recommended Response] to prevent [Health Threat].

1	2	3	4	5	6	7
Strongly Disagree						Strongly Agree

5. It is easy to [Perform Recommended Response] to prevent [Health Threat].

1	2	3	4	5	6	7
Strongly Disagree						Strongly Agree

6. I can [Perform Recommended Response] to prevent [Health Threat].

1	2	3	4	5	6	7
Strongly Disagree						Strongly Agree

Susceptibility

---

7. I am at risk for [Getting/Experiencing Health Threat].

1	2	3	4	5	6	7
Strongly Disagree						Strongly Agree

8. It is possible that I will [Get/Experience Health Threat].

1	2	3	4	5	6	7
Strongly Disagree						Strongly Agree

9. I am susceptible to [Getting/Experiencing Health Threat].

1	2	3	4	5	6	7
Strongly Disagree						Strongly Agree

Severity

---

10. [Health Threat] is a serious threat.

1	2	3	4	5	6	7
Strongly Disagree						Strongly Agree

11. [Health Threat] is harmful.

1	2	3	4	5	6	7
Strongly Disagree						Strongly Agree

12. [Health Threat] is a severe threat.

1	2	3	4	5	6	7
Strongly Disagree						Strongly Agree

Note: The specific items on the scale may be modified to fit the topic and audience of the health risk message under development.

threat items together. Fifth, subtract the threat score from the efficacy score. This number is your discriminating value.[1] Following is the simple formula you follow to determine the discriminating value.

$$\begin{aligned}
&(\Sigma \text{ Perceived Efficacy}) \\
-\ &\underline{(\Sigma \text{ Perceived Threat})} \\
=\ &\text{Discriminating Value (discriminates between fear control and danger control)}
\end{aligned}$$

where

Σ = sum of (i.e., add up all the items measuring perceived efficacy or perceived threat).

Your discriminating value is either a positive or negative number. A positive value means that your client or target audience is engaging in danger control processes because perceptions of efficacy are stronger than perceptions of threat. Thus, your client or target audience is likely to be engaging in some level of protective behaviors with regard to your specified health threat. A negative value means your client or target audience is engaging in fear control processes because perceptions of threat are stronger than perceptions of efficacy. Thus, your clients or target audience are likely to be engaging in fear control processes and are probably not protecting themselves against the specified health threat. Now that you know where your audience stands in terms of danger control or fear control, you can develop the most appropriate health risk message for them.

To summarize, all you do is add up the numbers circled for the efficacy items (i.e., the response efficacy and self-efficacy items) and the numbers circled for the threat items (i.e., the susceptibility and severity items) separately. For example, say for items 1 to 6 in Table 6.1 (the efficacy items) "4" was circled for each. For items 7 to 12 in Table 6.1 (the threat items), "5" was circled for each. Then, the sum of efficacy items (items 1 to 6) is 24 (4 + 4 + 4 + 4 + 4 + 4 = 24) and the sum of threat items (items 7 to 12) is 30 (5 + 5 + 5 + 5 + 5 + 5 = 30). Then, subtract the threat sum from the efficacy sum. Using the numbers above, the result is 24–30 =–6. The result is your "discriminating value" and in this case is a (–) negative number. Because our discriminating value is –6, a negative number, the person who responded to the questions on this scale was manifesting fear control regarding the health threat. If the final value had been positive, then this person would have been in danger control.

Once you have the discriminating value, you can develop on-the-spot messages that work for that particular person or audience. If the discriminating value is negative, use Message Type I below. If the discriminating value is positive, use Message Type II. If your client's or audience's answers to Table 6.1 and the threat items (items 7 to 12) all seem low (the numerals 1 or 2 most often circled), then use Message Type III. The following information provides a rationale for using these Message Types given differences in your discriminating value as well as the messages themselves.

■■ TAILORED HEALTH RISK MESSAGES

Recall that according to the EPPM, we want to move people toward high levels of danger control processing. To do this, individuals need to have high perceptions of threat and efficacy. When individuals or audiences have a negative discriminating value score, indicating they are engaging in fear control processes, then health risk messages that are too threatening may backfire. Alternatively, when people have a positive score, indicating they are in danger control, they may need threatening messages to motivate them to further action. In addition to looking at the overall discriminating value score, examine the scores for threat (items 7 to 12) and efficacy (items 1 to 6) individually as well as for each dimension of threat and efficacy (i.e., the response efficacy score, items 1 to 3; the self- efficacy score, items 4 to 6; the susceptibility score, items 7 to 9; and the severity score, items 10 to 12).

For example, if overall perceived efficacy is low, then an examination of the different dimension scores (i.e., the response efficacy dimension versus the self-efficacy dimension) tells you whether perceived response efficacy was low, perceived self-efficacy was low, or both efficacy dimensions were low. This information provides clues as to the variables needing emphasis in your health risk message. For example, if perceptions of response efficacy, self-efficacy, and severity are all high, but the individual has a very low susceptibility score, then you need to emphasize susceptibility issues for that person. You need to make them believe they are at risk and vulnerable to the threat. Following are specific types of messages that should be used depending on whether a negative or positive discriminating value results from the scale. A third message type is offered for individuals with low threat perceptions.

Message Type I: Negative Discriminating Value Scores
Indicating Dominance of Fear Control Process

For people with negative discriminating value scores, health risk messages must focus on increasing their perceptions of self-efficacy and response efficacy toward the recommended response. Because perceived threat is already high for these people, they should not be frightened further. Every attempt should be made to avoid references to the seriousness of the health threat or susceptibility to it. In fact, threatening messages to those in fear control, that is, with negative discriminating value scores, are likely to backfire and cause these people to put themselves at even greater risk for the health threat. In one study, we found that when people with low efficacy perceptions were made to feel susceptible to HIV/AIDS, they reported six weeks later that they slept around more and used condoms less! These people did the opposite of what the message advocated—the message backfired (Witte, 1991).

People in fear control need health risk messages that increase their perceptions of efficacy. Thus, these health risk messages should focus on response and self-efficacy issues regarding the recommended response. To increase response efficacy, practitioners or providers should emphasize the recommended response works and is effective in averting the threat or decreasing the chances of experiencing the health threat. For example, in the case of HIV/AIDS as the health threat and condoms as the recommended response, the emphasis should be on the fact that condoms decrease the chance of contracting sexually transmitted diseases and concrete examples of this statement should be provided.

Perceived self-efficacy often is more difficult to influence, especially if people already have low perceived efficacy. For example, in the case of condom use, many people may not believe they are actually capable of using condoms because they are too embarrassed to talk about them, fear that suggesting the use of a condom would ruin an intimate mood, or do not know how to bring up the topic in a sexual encounter. As outlined in chapter 4, Bandura (1977) notes that an individual's self-efficacy perceptions are developed from four sources of information: performance accomplishments (e.g., role playing, participant modeling), verbal persuasion (e.g., self-instruction, suggestion), vicarious experience (e.g., watching live or symbolic modeling), and physiological

CHAPTER 6

states (e.g., relaxation, biofeedback, and symbolic desensitization). Performance accomplishments, such as role-playing (or performing) the recommended behavior, often work very well in increasing self-efficacy perceptions. When people have the opportunity to role-play difficult behaviors or recommended responses, it provides them with ideas and strategies for how to act in real situations. Role-playing is especially useful for increasing perceived self-efficacy regarding a recommended response. The audience or clients might practice (a) bringing up the issue of condoms, (b) persuading a reluctant partner, and (c) persuading a willing partner to follow through on the use of condoms. If mass media are used, then actors similar to the target audience can role-play these same scenarios, providing the audience with a vicarious experience.

Message Type II: Positive Discriminating Values
Indicating Dominance of Danger Control Processes

People in danger control have sufficiently high perceptions of efficacy to counteract their threat perceptions. Thus, to continue motivating these people to engage in self-protective behaviors, health risk messages should emphasize the severity of the threat and the audiences' or clients' susceptibility to it. Most important, strong response efficacy and self-efficacy messages similar to those outlined above for people in fear control should accompany the high threat messages to ensure the efficacy level remains higher than the threat level. To increase perceived severity of the threat, vivid and intense language should be used to describe its consequences. For example, to increase perceived severity for genital warts (one of the most common sexually transmitted diseases on college campuses), it might be emphasized that such warts can cause bleeding, itching, and oozing, and grow so large as to block the birth canal (Fletcher, 1991; *HPV in perspective*, 1991). Furthermore, you might point out that genital warts are associated with cervical cancer and can lead to severe birth complications, such as when warty growths develop in the respiratory track of infants and lead to disability or even death (Fletcher, 1991; Knowles, 1994). These last two sentences paint a vivid picture regarding the severity of genital warts.

To increase perceived susceptibility toward a health threat, messages need to emphasize or illustrate how the health threat occurs in people who are demographically, psychographically, and in any other way possible, identical to your intended audiences or clients. Chapter 5 gave specific instructions on how to gather this information. One of the most effective ways to increase perceived susceptibility is to have someone adversely affected by the health threat who is similar to the intended audience speak to this audience live. In the case of genital warts, someone who has had great difficulty with genital warts (e.g., they've been painful, continue to grow back after treatment) and is very similar to the target audience (e.g., college student, has had only two sexual partners, serial monogamist) might talk candidly about how he or she failed to protect himself or herself, was not promiscuous, and contracted the warts from a girlfriend or boyfriend he or she trusted. Then, he or she should discuss the seriousness of genital warts and how they have affected his or her life. Similar health messages can be developed for mass media (see for example, Roberto, Meyer, Atkin, & Johnson, 2000).

These threatening messages help motivate your audience to further action. However, it is critical that threatening messages be accompanied by strong response and self-efficacy messages regarding the recommended response. You do not want to risk increasing threat perceptions to the point they begin to exceed efficacy perceptions because this would cause people to go into fear control. However, it is also important to judiciously use threatening messages to help to motivate people into far more action than efficacy-alone messages can.

*Message Type III: People with Low Threat
Perceptions (low scores for items 7 to 12)*

People with low threat perceptions are likely to have a danger control discriminating value score, even with their low efficacy perceptions. For example, if individuals respond with a "1" to all the perceived threat items (indicating low perceived threat) and "1" or "2" to all the perceived efficacy items (indicating low perceived efficacy), their efficacy score still outweighs their threat score to produce a discriminating value indicating danger control dominance. It is useful to examine the threat portion of the scale to determine if the audiences or clients lack perceived susceptibility, perceived severity, or both.

For example, if the threat score is 12 or less, then audiences or clients most likely have low threat perceptions (i.e., meaning they chose 1 or 2 as responses for the six items measuring perceptions of severity and susceptibility). Or perhaps they responded with a "1" for susceptibility but "6" or "7" for severity. If so, their responses indicate they have high severity but low susceptibility perceptions. Thus, these people may think the threat is severe (such as HIV/AIDS) but don't think they are susceptible to it. Or, sometimes people think they are susceptible to a threat (choosing 6 or 7) but think the threat is trivial or harmless (choosing 1 or 2 for the severity items). Health risk messages can then be constructed accordingly to directly influence these severity perceptions, susceptibility perceptions, or both.

For people with low perceptions of threat, danger control messages such as those outlined earlier in this chapter are most appropriate. People with low perceived threat need to be convinced of the seriousness of the health threat and their susceptibility to it, as well as the ease and feasibility of the recommended responses. It is especially important to break through the invulnerability barriers with high perceived susceptibility messages for these people. Again, it is critical that any attempt to increase perceptions of threat be accompanied by messages increasing perceptions of efficacy as well.

Summary of Message Types

In sum, a positive discriminating value score indicates that to be effective, health risk messages should outline risks, hazards, and the harmful effects of a particular threat, as well as describe effective responses to avert the threats. This type of high threat/high efficacy message motivates further action. In contrast, a negative discriminating value score indicates that effective health risk messages should emphasize the ability to perform the recommended responses, as well as the effectiveness and ease of the recommended responses in averting a health threat. Little, if any, reference should be made to the threat. For those individuals with low perceived threat, special attention should be paid to increasing their perceptions of severity and susceptibility.

∎ SOME ADDITIONAL GUIDELINES

If you are assessing a discriminating value for an entire audience, then the procedure you follow is a bit different. Instead of giving the scale to an individual client, you give it to a random sample of the target audience. Then, average your audience's responses and analyze them as a whole to determine the best type of message for them. For example, say you have a sample of 10 people from your target audience. Their discriminating values are 2, –2, 5, 1, 3, –1, 4, 5, 3, and 6. To average these discriminating values, simply add them up and divide by 10 (the total number of people in your sample). Therefore, the average discriminating value for this sample is +2.6 [(2 + –2 + 5 + 1 + 3 + –1 + 4 + 5 + 3 + 6 = 26)/10 = 2.6].

Overall, when determining audience discriminating values you should look at two things. First, average the individual scores given by members of your target audience into one overall score (as described in the preceding paragraph). The average is either positive or negative. If it's positive, then your audience as a whole is in danger control; if it's negative, then your audience as a whole is in fear control.

However, when averaging scores, it's important to examine the individual discriminating value scores given by members of your target audience as well. If you notice one or two extremely high or extremely low scores, then you may wish to re-average the scores without these people's responses. Those "outlying" scores may be skewing the results. Second, look at everyone's discriminating value score individually and tally how many were positive (i.e., indicating danger control with regard to the threat) and how many were negative (i.e., indicating fear control with regard to the threat). For example, you may find that out of a sample of 30 members of your target audience, 23 had positive scores and seven had negative scores. If both the audience average and the tally of individual scores match (i.e., both positive scores or both negative scores), then you can be fairly confident you have an accurate estimate of whether your audience is in danger control or fear control. However, if the numbers don't match—for example, your average is positive but when you tally up individual responses 25 people had negative scores and only five people had positive scores—then you need to check for outliers or extreme responses. It is important to determine why the numbers don't match. Once you have determined whether individuals are in fear control or danger control, then you can develop an effective risk message that targets the overall beliefs and perceptions of your audience.

■■ CONCLUSION

Knowing your audience or clients' threat and efficacy perceptions is key to the development of effective health risk messages because it allows you to develop on-the-spot, targeted messages addressing specific perceptions of threat and efficacy. Overall, the RBD Scale was developed because health risk messages targeted toward someone who is currently engaging in "no response" need to be very different from messages aimed at someone engaging in fear control or danger control responses. Once trained in how to use the scale, you can make judgments about your audience or clients' current perceptions of threat and efficacy and develop effective health risk messages in just a minute or two. The next chapter gives real-life examples on how to use the scale.

■■ NOTE

1. In older versions of the RBD Scale, we standardized (i.e., converted to Z-scores) the threat scores and the efficacy scores before summing them. However, research showed that there was little, if any, difference between using raw scores and Z-scores. Therefore, for simplicity, we have presented the raw score version of the scale, which people are more likely to use.

7

Out of the Tower
and Into the Field

This chapter offers several examples of how the RBD Scale is used in the HIV Counseling and Testing Program at the campus health center of Michigan State University. Remember, the RBD Scale can be used for any health topic or recommended response; we're showing you just one application of the strategies outlined in this book. The RBD Scale has been used at the campus health center since the spring of 1995 by a team of HIV counselors and testers led by one of the authors. He compares the RBD Scale to a mechanic's tool. As he explains,

> My father was a mechanic who had a seemingly magical box filled with wonderful tools. As a child, I was amazed at how he could utilize those tools to diagnose and/or fix just about any automobile that entered his garage. When I turned 10, I received a new monkey wrench as a birthday present. I was so excited with my very own tool that I went about looking for something to work on. I remembered that my bicycle needed to have the seat adjusted so I thought I'd take care of it with my new tool! Before long I had stripped the bolt, was completely frustrated, and had to go find good ol' dad to fix things. My father surveyed the situation and proceeded to fix the problem. As he finished he left me with these words of wisdom: "Son, a tool does not make you a mechanic. Using a tool takes a thorough understanding of how it works, what it is used for, and an understanding of what you will use it on." He added, "Combine this knowledge with practice and patience and you will be an able mechanic."

The author thinks the RBD Scale (his tool) has increased his precision in diagnosing why his clients may or may not be protecting themselves against HIV infection. He also believes "the tool," as he calls the RBD Scale, has increased his effectiveness in promoting safer sex behaviors dramatically. At the same time, he believes that like a mechanic, practitioners need a thorough understanding of the concepts and theory behind the RBD Scale (the tool) to solve problems and use it effectively.

■■ USING THE RBD SCALE AT A CAMPUS HEALTH CLINIC: BACKGROUND

The HIV Counseling, Testing, and Referral (CTR) program at Michigan State University was the setting for a pilot application and then full adoption of the Risk Behavior Diagnosis Scale. The HIV-CTR program is housed in the campus health center, which services students, faculty, staff, and, in limited cases, the public. The program counsels and tests approximately 500 to 700 clients per year. The clients range in age from 17 to 54, with the mean age being 21. The program and counselors are certified and trained by the Michigan Department of Community Health (MDCH) and the Centers for Disease Control and Prevention (CDC).

In 1994, the CDC shifted its counseling philosophy and began requiring all designated testing sites to use the "client-centered" approach to counseling, testing, and referral. The new model was based on health behavior change theory. Under this model, a counselor was required to do prevention counseling as opposed to test counseling. In prevention counseling, a counselor

- provides the client with the opportunity to assist in identifying his or her risk of acquiring or transmitting HIV
- provides the client with an opportunity to negotiate and reinforce a plan to reduce or eliminate risk
- translates the client's risk perception into a risk reduction plan that may be enhanced by knowledge of HIV infection status
- helps the client initiate and sustain behavior changes to reduce the risks of acquiring or transmitting HIV (CDC, 1994)

In test counseling, by contrast, a counselor merely disseminates the results of an HIV test and provides information on where to seek help if the result is positive.

With the transition from test counseling to prevention counseling, the primary goal of counseling has now become behavior change. Under the client-centered model, the counselor is expected to "assess the client's readiness to adopt safer behaviors by identifying behavior changes the client has already implemented and negotiate a realistic and incremental plan for reducing risk" (CDC, 1994). The counselor now is expected to work with clients to determine ways to help them make self-protective behavior changes. Unfortunately, although HIV counselors and testers were given this mandate, they were not provided with specific theoretical guidance concerning the best way to promote behavior change in clients. It appears that many, if not most, practitioners fail to systematically develop risk-reduction messages based on some sort of theoretical guidance. In fact, a survey of HIV service providers found that the vast majority of practitioners in this sample "discounted theory" and did not use it when developing risk-reduction messages (Dearing et al., 1996). However, as we have pointed out in this book, using theory to guide message development not only makes the job easier but also increases effectiveness.

The majority of clients who use the HIV-CTR service at the health center register for their appointments anonymously. A unique ID number is issued to clients when they register. In addition, clients must pick up educational materials and two paper-and-pencil assessments to complete before they arrive for their appointments. Clients are instructed to read the materials and fill out the forms.

Of the two forms clients complete before seeing a counselor, one is an educational assessment and the other is a combination of an HIV risk/background assessment and the Risk Behavior Diagnosis Scale (Table 7.1). Notice that the RBD Scale was placed at the end of the form and does not include scoring diagrams or information. This was done to alleviate any scoring anxiety clients might experience when answering the questions. The counselors were instructed to score the RBD items without visibly making calculations on the sheet.

We have found that, with practice, a counselor can look at the pattern of answers to the questions and immediately determine if the person is engaging in danger or fear control processes without the need to numerically figure the score. We have found that using the scale without scoring it is relatively easy. You simply memorize the fact that the first six items are efficacy items and the last six items are threat items. If the first six items have higher scores than the last six, you know the person is in danger control (because the first six items representing efficacy are higher than the next six items representing threat). If the last six items have higher scores than the first six items, then you know the person is in fear control (because the six items representing threat are scored higher than the six items representing efficacy). For example, look at the following RBD responses from Hannah and Dylan. Can you tell by simply scanning their responses who is in fear control and who is in danger control?

Hannah's RBD Responses

	Strongly Disagree				Strongly Agree
1. Using condoms is effective in preventing AIDS.	1	2	3	④	5
2. Condoms work in preventing AIDS.	1	2	3	4	⑤
3. If I use a condom, I am less likely to get AIDS.	1	2	3	4	⑤
4. Using condoms to prevent AIDS is convenient.	1	2	3	4	⑤
5. Using condoms to prevent AIDS is easy.	1	2	3	④	5
6. I am able to use condoms to prevent getting AIDS.	1	2	3	④	5
7. I believe that AIDS is severe.	1	②	3	4	5
8. I believe that AIDS is a significant disease.	1	2	③	4	5
9. I believe that AIDS is serious.	1	②	3	4	5
10. It is likely that I will contract AIDS.	①	2	3	4	5
11. I am at risk for getting AIDS.	①	2	3	4	5
12. It is possible that I will contract AIDS.	1	②	3	4	5

Dylan's RBD Responses

	Strongly Disagree				Strongly Agree
1. Using condoms is effective in preventing AIDS.	1	②	3	4	5
2. Condoms work in preventing AIDS.	1	②	3	4	5
3. If I use a condom, I am less likely to get AIDS.	1	②	3	4	5
4. Using condoms to prevent AIDS is convenient.	1	2	③	4	5
5. Using condoms to prevent AIDS is easy.	①	2	3	4	5
6. I am able to use condoms to prevent getting AIDS.	①	2	3	4	5
7. I believe that AIDS is severe.	1	2	3	4	⑤
8. I believe that AIDS is a significant disease.	1	2	3	4	⑤
9. I believe that AIDS is serious.	1	2	3	4	⑤
10. It is likely that I will contract AIDS.	1	2	3	④	5
11. I am at risk for getting AIDS.	1	2	3	④	5
12. It is possible that I will contract AIDS.	1	2	3	4	⑤

CHAPTER 7

Table 7.1   Risk & Background Assessments, RBD Scale

Olin Health Center: Center for Sexual Health Promotion

Please complete this form and bring it with you to your Pre-test Counseling session. Completing this survey helps to facilitate the process. Your responses are confidential—DO NOT PUT YOUR NAME ANYWHERE ON THIS FORM. If you are uncomfortable completing the form or don't understand something, your provider will discuss and complete it with you during your appointment. You may also write down additional questions or concerns you want to discuss.

BACKGROUND INFORMATION

What is your sex? _____ Female _____ Male
What is your age? _____

Please rate your anxiety level about being tested.
_____ High
_____ Moderate
_____ Low
_____ Very low
_____ Very high

Are you requesting an _____ anonymous or
_____ confidential test?

WHY ARE YOU REQUESTING HIV TESTING?
Please mark all possible reasons that may apply:
_____ I was sexually assaulted.
_____ I'm curious about my HIV status because of some doubts about past partner(s).
_____ I'm contemplating a new relationship and "want to be sure" I won't transmit HIV.
_____ My current partner asked me to have the test.
_____ My values and/or priorities have changed and I'm trying to rectify past decisions.
_____ I've recently been diagnosed with another STD.
_____ I've been exhibiting symptoms for HIV infection or AIDS. Please list symptoms:_____
_____ This test is the recommended follow-up to a previous test.
_____ I'm traveling to another country and the test is required.
_____ The test is required for my application to Peace Corps, military service, or other job.
_____ I've had a partner tell me that s/he has tested positive for HIV and/or an STD.
_____ I've had a health department, doctor or other medical care professional, blood bank, drug treatment service, or other agency recommend that I be tested.
_____ I've been occupationally exposed to blood/body fluids.
_____ I have potentially exposed a medical care worker and was asked to be tested.
_____ I'm getting married and was motivated by a premarital certification class.
_____ I'm thinking of becoming (or am) pregnant and want to be able to make plans.
_____ I've recently been diagnosed with tuberculosis.
Other reason(s):_____

POTENTIAL RISK(S) FOR HIV INFECTION
Please mark all potential risks that may apply:
_____ I've had sex with males.
_____ I've had sex with females.
_____ I've used injecting drugs. If marked, please list the drug(s): _____
_____ I've had sex while under the influence of (circle all that apply): alcohol, marijuana, PCP, speed, crack cocaine, Cocaine, heroin, opiates.
_____ I've given or received drugs and/or money in exchange for sex.
_____ I've been diagnosed with an STD.
_____ I've had sex with an injecting drug user.
_____ I've had sex with a man who has had sex with another man.
_____ I've had sex with a person with HIV/AIDS.
_____ I've had sex with a person who received blood and/or blood products.
_____ I've had sex with a person who was at other risk for HIV. Describe the risk: _____
_____ I have a bleeding disorder that requires therapy with clotting factor or other blood products.
_____ I received blood/blood products between 1978 and 1985.
_____ I was exposed to blood/body fluids in a health care setting or at the scene of an accident.
_____ I've been sexually assaulted.
Other risks: _____

Please think about how you might respond to the following questions that your provider may discuss with you. You *do not need to write* out your responses.

When was your last potential risk?
    How would a positive result affect your life? What might you do differently, what changes might you make?
    How would a negative result affect your life? What might you do differently, what changes might you make?
    How do you plan to deal with any anxiety or stress you may experience while waiting two weeks for your test results?
    How do you plan to reduce your risk of acquiring or transmitting HIV in the future?

For each of the following statements, please indicate how much you agree or disagree by circling the appropriate response on a scale of 1 to 5, where "1" means "strongly disagree" and "5" means "strongly agree."

	Strongly Disagree				Strongly Agree
1. Using condoms is effective in preventing AIDS.	1	2	3	4	5
2. Condoms work in preventing AIDS.	1	2	3	4	5
3. If I use a condom, I am less likely to get AIDS.	1	2	3	4	5
4. Using condoms to prevent AIDS is convenient.	1	2	3	4	5
5. Using condoms to prevent AIDS is easy.	1	2	3	4	5
6. I am able to use condoms to prevent getting AIDS.	1	2	3	4	5
7. I believe AIDS is severe.	1	2	3	4	5
8. I believe that AIDS is a significant disease.	1	2	3	4	5
9. I believe that AIDS is serious.	1	2	3	4	5
10. It is likely that I will contract AIDS.	1	2	3	4	5
11. I am at risk for getting AIDS.	1	2	3	4	5
12. It is possible that I will contract AIDS.	1	2	3	4	5

Thank you for completing this form, *please be sure to bring it with you to your appointment!!*

By quickly reviewing the responses, you can tell that Hannah scored high on items 1 to 6 (efficacy) and low on items 7 to 12 (threat). Because you know items 1 to 6 reflect efficacy perceptions and items 7 to 12 reflect threat perceptions you can tell with a glance that Hannah has higher efficacy perceptions than threat perceptions. And, you also know that when efficacy perceptions are higher than threat perceptions, the person is in danger control. Therefore, you now know Hannah is in danger control regarding HIV infection and needs to be motivated to act through messages that increase her perceived severity of AIDS and her perceived susceptibility to HIV infection. In other words, Hannah's scores indicate that she knows she can protect herself against HIV infection (i.e., perceived self-efficacy) and she believes that condoms work in preventing HIV infection (i.e., perceived response efficacy), but she doesn't believe that AIDS is a very serious disease (i.e., perceived severity) and she doesn't believe that she is at risk for HIV infection (i.e., perceived susceptibility). Therefore according to the EPPM, to promote behavior change, the counselor needs to emphasize the seriousness of HIV/AIDS to Hannah and convince her of her vulnerability to infection if she engages in unsafe sexual practices.

Now, take a look at Dylan's scores and estimate whether he's in danger control or fear control. By reviewing his responses, you can tell his efficacy perceptions toward condoms are low (items 1 to 6) and his threat perceptions are high (items 7 to 12). You know when perceived threat exceeds perceived efficacy, fear control processes dominate. Therefore, because Dylan's threat scores are higher than his efficacy scores, you know he's in fear control. He needs messages emphasizing the effectiveness of condoms in deterring HIV infection (i.e., response efficacy) as well as messages increasing his perceived ability to use condoms (i.e., self-efficacy). In terms of the latter, it is important to find out why Dylan does not see himself as able to use condoms to prevent HIV infection and then address each of his concerns in turn.

After you have used the scale 20 or 30 times, you can easily "score" the scale automatically. After you have learned to automatically score the RBD, you can also examine the individual dimensions of response efficacy, self-efficacy, severity, and susceptibility, and address each of these specifically in your message. All you need to do is memorize that the items 1 to 3 represent response efficacy; items 4 to 6 represent self-efficacy; items 7 to 9 represent severity; and items 10 to 12 represent susceptibility. If a person scores high on all items except items 7 to 9, then you know this person needs to be convinced of the severity of AIDS because items 7 to 9 deal with the perceived seriousness of the health threat.

Examining the RBD Scale for consistent patterns is helpful to practitioners in two ways. First, they can quickly discern how to proceed with the prevention messages. Second, any individual items that are scored substantially differently from the overall pattern of responses can be used to further "diagnose" problem perceptions or issues. Also, responses that differ from the general pattern can be used as checkpoints to determine whether the client understood the questions in the scale.

HIV counseling and testing is very intense and emotional and of a short duration. Most counselors can offer no more than 30 minutes per client. In that time frame, clients must be assessed for their potential risks of HIV infection, allowed to ask any questions they might have, provided instructions for filling out forms, sent down for a blood or saliva collection, assessed for readiness to adopt safer behaviors, and given messages to help initiate and sustain behavior changes to reduce their risks. As you can see, any tool that quickly helps a counselor determine the most effective way to promote protective behaviors is needed and useful.

In the following section are four case studies of individuals who presented themselves for HIV counseling and testing at the campus health center. The survey appearing in Table 7.1 was completed prior to their appointments. The HIV counselor reviewed each part of the survey, examining the RBD Scale last. Once the RBD Scale was reviewed, then either (a) message construction began or (b) further questions were formulated to diagnose exactly the perceptions contributing to a client's fear or danger control state. The recommended response for the clients at this HIV clinic was condoms for the following reasons:

1. the majority of the clients (90%) presenting at this clinic give unprotected sex as their major risk factor and the reason for being tested;

2. nearly all of the clients were gay or heterosexual (i.e., bisexual and trans-sexual clients were rare); and

3. condoms are easily obtained and theoretically simple to use.

The process of HIV counseling and testing often produces extreme anxiety in clients. This anxiety can cause the client either to be very receptive to health messages or very defensive against messages. It is incumbent upon the counselor to evaluate clients' anxiety level to determine the timing of the message. For some clients, the messages can be delivered during the precounseling session; for others it may be prudent to wait until the results have been given at the postcounseling session. When messages are given at the precounseling session, they should be reinforced in the postcounseling session. The timing of delivering a message is very important. With practice you can sense when a client is most receptive to hearing a health risk message.

CASE ONE

Bob (not his real name) was a heterosexual male who presented himself for HIV counseling and testing with "unprotected intercourse with a female under the influence of alcohol" as his only risk. This was his first test. After reviewing the assessment materials the counselor examined Bob's RBD Scale (Table 7.2.).[1]

The first three questions dealt with Bob's beliefs about whether condoms were actually effective as a risk-reduction method (i.e., response efficacy). In reviewing the responses to the first three questions, you see that the client responded with "5" (Strongly Agree) to all of them. This indicates the client believes condoms are effective as a means of preventing HIV infection. Bob also responded with "5" (Strongly Agree) to each item on the second component of the efficacy scale (questions 3 to 6), which assessed his beliefs regarding his ability to utilize the recommended response (self-efficacy). These scores indicate that Bob believes he is easily able to use condoms to prevent HIV infection.

Upon seeing these scores, the counselor initiated dialogue by probing further into each topic.

Counselor: I see you believe condoms are an effective way to reduce your risk.

Bob: Yeah, everyone says so.

Table 7.2   Case One (Bob)

For each of the following statements, please indicate how much you agree or disagree by circling the appropriate response on a scale of 1 to 5, where "1" means "strongly disagree" and "5" means "strongly agree."

	Strongly Disagree				Strongly Agree	
1. Using condoms is effective in preventing AIDS.	1	2	3	4	(5)	
2. Condoms work in preventing AIDS.	1	2	3	4	(5)	ΣRE = 15
3. If I use a condom, I am less likely to get AIDS.	1	2	3	4	(5)	
4. Using condoms to prevent AIDS is convenient.	1	2	3	4	(5)	
5. Using condoms to prevent AIDS is easy.	1	2	3	4	(5)	ΣSE = 15
6. I am able to use condoms to prevent getting AIDS.	1	2	3	4	(5)	
						ΣEFFICACY = 30
7. I believe that AIDS is severe.	1	2	3	4	(5)	
8. I believe AIDS is a significant disease.	1	2	3	4	(5)	ΣSEV = 15
9. I believe that AIDS is serious.	1	2	3	4	(5)	
10. It is likely that I will contract AIDS.	1	(2)	3	4	5	
11. I am at risk for getting AIDS.	1	(2)	3	4	5	ΣSUSC = 8
12. It is possible that I will contract AIDS.	1	2	3	(4)	5	
						ΣTHREAT = 23
			DISCRIMINATING VALUE		+7	

Counselor: Do you always use condoms when you have sex?

Bob: Well, when I had a girlfriend, we started off using condoms but as time went on she started the pill. We only broke up about three weeks ago so I haven't had a chance to get more condoms and I didn't think I'd be using them so soon.

Asking questions like these about each topic helps spot-check the client's answers. Be alert to signs of hesitation and/or doubt. If you sense hesitation or doubt, probe further to ensure that the client answered the questions based on his or her true beliefs. Sometimes clients answer questions in the way they think they should, instead of based on what they truly believe. The counselor continued his probing, alert to the fact that something different happened during the last three weeks.

Counselor: What happened during the last three weeks?

Bob: I was out at a local bar about two weeks ago on bar night (what Thursday night is called at Michigan State University) with some friends and my former girlfriend was there making a complete idiot of herself. She had a new boyfriend who had his hands all over her and she was looking like she enjoyed it. Some girl kept hitting on me, so finally I got up and danced with her. I wanted to show my old girlfriend that she wasn't the only one who was attractive to other people. I got wasted that night and made sure I left before my old girlfriend did and I made sure that she saw me leaving with this girl hanging all over me. I barely remember doing it but I know that I didn't use a condom. The next day I felt really stupid and all my friends told me that this girl has slept with all kinds of weirdos —including me now, I guess. My friends tell me I was being a real jerk. I don't really think I've gotten AIDS from her, but I thought I'd rather be safe than sorry, so I made this appointment.

The counselor then examined the part of the scale that measured threat severity (7 to 9). Once again, the client responded with "5" (Strongly agree) to all the items, indicating he believes AIDS is a severe threat. At this point, the counselor makes one of two judgments:

1. The client's perception of the threat is high enough and the severity of AIDS does not need to be emphasized in a message.

2. Test anxiety has influenced Bob to exaggerate his perception of severity. Keep in mind that test anxiety, individuals' propensity to respond to questions in a socially desirable way (i.e., they want to present themselves in a positive manner), and/or demand characteristics (i.e., when people respond the way they think they should, but not the way they really feel), can influence how people respond to the scale. That's why it is useful to probe further into some topics.

In terms of his susceptibility to threat, Bob scored considerably lower (2,2,4). These scores indicate he has a relatively low perception of susceptibility toward the threat. In our experience, the susceptibility to threat portion of the scale is where you find the most variation in scores. Most people do not want to believe they are at risk for given health threats, especially AIDS. Given Bob's disclosure about having unprotected sex under the influence of alcohol, and the fact that Bob indicated this was a rare occurrence, the counselor decided not to ask further questions about the susceptibility scores. The counselor also noted that according to Bob's survey, he did not appear to be engaging in high-risk activities, save this isolated incident, nor did he appear to be a member of a high-risk demographic group. Therefore, the counselor decided to move straight into scoring the full scale and developing preventive messages.

Bob scored a total of 30 out of 30 on the efficacy portion of the scale and a total of 23 out of 30 for the threat portion of the scale (15 on severity and 8 on susceptibility). Using the formula provided in Chapter 6, in which threat scores are subtracted from efficacy scores to yield a discriminating value, Bob's discriminating value is calculated to be +7 (i.e., 30 − 23 = 7). This score indicates Bob has sufficiently high perceptions of efficacy to counteract his threat perceptions. Therefore, he should be engaging in danger control processes, according to the RBD Scale. Indeed, the fact that Bob appeared for counseling and testing based on a single unsafe sexual incident indicates he is attempting to protect himself against the threat of HIV—a danger control action.

Based on the +7 danger control score, the counselor decided Bob needed motivation to use condoms to prevent HIV infection, no matter what the scenario, as he already believed he was effectively able to use condoms to prevent HIV infection. The counselor also believed Bob's assessment of his susceptibility to the threat of HIV infection was fairly accurate; Bob reported engaging in only one high-risk sexual activity and seemed to use condoms on other occasions. The counselor recognized Bob's recent breakup with his girlfriend, an emotionally devastating event, appeared to contribute to the unsafe sex incident. However, the counselor wanted to ensure Bob did not repeat this alcohol and unsafe sex episode.

Therefore, the counselor developed the health risk message according to the following factors:

1. Bob was engaging in danger control processes, given the +7 discriminating value, indicating that threat issues needed to be emphasized to motivate action and efficacy perceptions needed to be reinforced.

2. Based on the efficacy probe, the counselor determined Bob needed more immediate access to condoms.

3. Bob scored the maximum possible on the three items measuring threat severity, indicating that he was already convinced of the severity of HIV infection.

4. Bob scored relatively low on the three items measuring susceptibility to the threat, indicating that he needed to be convinced he was susceptible to contracting HIV.

5. Based on the probe, the counselor determined that the issue of unsafe sex under the influence of alcohol needed to be addressed, as did Bob's emotional state regarding his ex-girlfriend.

The counselor proceeded with his theoretically based preventive counseling by reinforcing the effectiveness of condoms as a preventive measure against HIV (i.e., reinforcing response efficacy); supporting Bob's belief that he was able to use condoms correctly to prevent infection (i.e., reinforcing self-efficacy), affirming that HIV infection and AIDS were indeed serious health problems (i.e., reinforcing severity of threat), and emphasizing his susceptibility to HIV infection when engaging in unprotected sex (i.e., increasing susceptibility to threat). As the following exchange illustrates, the counselor addressed each of the four theoretical constructs to promote strong perceptions of threat

CHAPTER 7

and efficacy to promote danger control outcomes such as self-protective behavior changes.

Counselor:	I see that you know AIDS is a serious disease and that you know how to use condoms to protect yourself against it.
Bob:	Yeah.
Counselor:	Do you ever have any problems using condoms or getting hold of them?
Bob:	No, I just didn't have any that night because I didn't think I'd need them. I guess I thought my girlfriend and I would get back together so I never even thought about getting any.
Counselor:	Do you have some now?
Bob:	No, I'm not interested in seeing anyone so I won't need them. I just want to make sure I'm clean.
Counselor:	It sounds like you weren't planning on seeing anyone that night either, but then you needed them. I have a bunch here if you want.
Bob:	OK, I know, I guess I'll take a few. Thanks.
Counselor:	You know how to use them?
Bob:	I've had plenty of practice; I just didn't have any that night.
Counselor:	You know, it's really dangerous to hook up with someone when you're drunk and have sex. The statistics show that lots of people just like you get HIV when they mix alcohol and unsafe sex. Would you do things differently next time?
Bob:	Yeah, I know it was stupid. That's why I came to get tested. I don't think it will happen again but if it does I've got these now (holds up condoms).
Counselor:	Good, I don't think there will be a next time either, but now you have condoms if there is. Have you talked with anyone about your breakup with your girlfriend?
Bob:	There's nothing to talk about. It's over. She made that perfectly clear.
Counselor:	Sometimes it helps to talk to a counselor about these things. Here's the name and number of someone who works here who might be able to help you (hands card of colleague).

This health risk message contained support for Bob's beliefs about condoms as effective protection against HIV (response efficacy), confirmed his effective use of condoms (self-efficacy), ensured he had access to them (gave him condoms), and addressed the underlying cause leading to unsafe sex (breakup with girlfriend, referred for counseling). There was no need to increase Bob's belief that AIDS was a severe threat according to the scale, and none was given. However, Bob received a very brief message concerning his cohort's susceptibility to HIV infection while under the influence of alcohol.

This case illustrates the usefulness of formative research prior to the delivery of an effective health risk message. In this case, the formative research was the precounseling survey and RBD Scale. Bob's responses to the formative survey indicated that he belonged to a group that demographically and behaviorally had a relatively low risk of HIV infection. Thus, trying to increase his perceived susceptibility to extremely high levels would have been deceitful and unwarranted, and may have led him to become what we call one of "the worried well," that is, people who seek health care unnecessarily.

CASE TWO

Jill (not her real name) was a 21-year-old heterosexual female who presented herself for HIV counseling and testing with unprotected intercourse under the influence of alcohol as her major risk factors. She had had several unprotected partners who had "ejaculated inside" of her. Most of these risks occurred while she was under the influence of alcohol. This was her first test and she was very anxious. After reviewing the rest of the materials, the counselor then turned to Jill's RBD Scale (Table 7.3).

In reviewing Jill's response efficacy score on the RBD Scale (items 1 to 3), you see she scores a modest 11 out of a possible 15. This indicates some inconsistencies in her beliefs concerning condoms as an effective risk-reduction response. Jill scored similarly low (10) on the items pertaining to self-efficacy (i.e., items 4 to 6). This score indicates that she questions her ability to use condoms to prevent HIV infection. The counselor took a quick look at the risk profile before beginning the session and found it indicated a lack of condom usage.

The counselor began his session by assessing the client's understanding of the questions and finding out more details about the relatively low efficacy scores.

Counselor: I can see by your answers that you're not entirely certain that condoms are effective.

Table 7.3 Case Two (Jill)

For each of the following statements, please indicate how much you agree or disagree by circling the appropriate response on a scale of 1 to 5, where "1" means "strongly disagree" and "5" means "strongly agree."

	Strongly Disagree				Strongly Agree	
1. Using condoms is effective in preventing AIDS.	1	2	③	4	5	
2. Condoms work in preventing AIDS.	1	2	③	4	5	ΣRE = 11
3. If I use a condom, I am less likely to get AIDS.	1	2	3	4	⑤	
4. Using condoms to prevent AIDS is convenient.	1	2	③	4	5	
5. Using condoms to prevent AIDS is easy.	1	2	③	4	5	ΣSE = 10
6. I am able to use condoms to prevent getting AIDS.	1	2	3	④	5	
						ΣEFFICACY = 21
7. I believe that AIDS is severe.	1	2	3	4	⑤	
8. I believe that AIDS is a significant disease.	1	2	3	4	⑤	ΣSEV = 5
9. I believe that AIDS is serious.	1	2	3	4	⑤	
10. It is likely that I will contract AIDS.	①	2	3	4	5	
11. I am at risk for getting AIDS.	1	2	3	④	5	ΣSUSC = 9
12. It is possible that I will contract AIDS.	1	2	3	④	5	
						ΣTHREAT = 24
				DISCRIMINATING VALUE	−3	

Jill: No, I guess not. I mean, sometimes you hear they work and sometimes you hear they don't.

Counselor: Have you ever used condoms?

Jill: Not really. I just think it'll make it feel different and I don't see how they can stay on. I once got that sponge birth control thing stuck inside me and almost had to go to the hospital to get it out. The last thing I want is to get a condom stuck up inside of me.

This exchange shows that Jill's perception of response and self-efficacy toward condoms is really based on a lack of experience using them. Her perceptions appear to be formed by what she had read and by analogies related to her experiences with another birth control device (e.g., the sponge) instead. The counselor then assessed the threat portion of the RBD Scale.

Jill predictably scored the highest on the three items measuring severity of threat (15). This is common for clients with this type of profile. We have found that female clients with low perceptions of response and self-efficacy, who utilize drugs (mainly alcohol) during sexual encounters, typically are driven into HIV counseling and testing by high perceptions of threat and feelings of fear.

Turning to susceptibility to threat, we see an inconsistent scoring pattern, with one score of 1 (Strongly Disagree), and two scores of 4 (toward Agree). This inconsistent pattern should raise a red flag in the professional's mind and be probed further.

Counselor: Why do you believe that you are not likely to contract AIDS (item 10 in Table 7.3), but you feel fairly strong that you are at risk for getting AIDS (items 11 and 12 in Table 7.3)?

Jill: Ummm . . . I know I'm at risk because I sometimes sleep with people without a condom and I don't know that much about them but I'm really scared about it, too. I don't want to admit to myself I really could get AIDS, so I always talk myself out of it.

Jill's honest answer revealed a remarkable self-awareness. She basically admitted she knew she was at risk given her behaviors, but also admitted she practiced denial techniques to manage her fear about contracting HIV. Whenever you see split scores such as these within the susceptibility portion of the RBD Scale, be sure to probe carefully by pointing out the inconsistencies to the client in a calm and low key manner. More often than not, clues are revealed about the clients' typical coping mechanisms for managing fearful events. Then, you can specifically address this coping style with your prevention message.

In terms of the overall RBD Scale, even with a relatively low susceptibility score, Jill's discriminating value score was -3 [(11 response efficacy + 10 self-efficacy = 21 efficacy) - (15 severity + 9 susceptibility = 24 threat) = -3]. This score indicates she is engaging in fear control processes. This finding is consistent with Jill's response to the question about the inconsistency in her susceptibility score. That is, it is clear Jill is very frightened of HIV infection, yet because of her inexperience with condoms, she did not feel able to do something to effectively avert the threat. So instead, she controlled her fear through denial strategies.

When composing the health risk message, the counselor made every effort to avoid references to the seriousness of the threat or to Jill's susceptibility to the threat for fear of pushing her further into fear control processes. Instead, the counselor focused on diminishing her anxiety by focusing on response and self-efficacy issues. In addition, the counselor attempted to reduce anxiety by giving factual information about Jill's susceptibility to HIV given her demographic and risk characteristics. For example, even with this client's risk factors, the epidemiological data points to a low prevalence among her cohort.

Great care must be taken when addressing the susceptibility issue. On the one hand, you need to reduce anxiety so the client can hear and act on recommended responses. On the other hand, you do not want to reduce perceived susceptibility to the point where clients believe they no longer need protection against the threat.

Counselor: First off, I want you to know that HIV infection is still relatively rare for people of your age and background. It's good that you came in to get tested so you can put your mind at ease. You do need to protect yourself, however, but the majority of people I see like you do not test positive for HIV. I think we need to make sure that this issue doesn't come up again, though. So, I think we need to talk about how you can protect yourself.

Jill: OK, I just don't think I can use condoms. All of my friends say when they use them they don't work anyway because they break or get holes in them.

Counselor: Well, let's start off by each opening a pack and seeing how elastic they are and just what it takes to break them.

The counselor then spent a great deal of time discussing the current literature and studies on condom effectiveness. He demonstrated the strength and durability of the condoms the health center provided. The counselor also showed how it would be extremely improbable for a condom to break during intercourse or have holes in it by blowing it up into a huge balloon. Following these response efficacy messages, the counselor turned to self-efficacy issues.

Creating and delivering messages to increase perceptions of self-efficacy can be difficult in a short period of time. As stated earlier, Bandura (1977) notes that an individual's perceptions of self-efficacy evolve from several sources of information, including vicarious and direct experience. In this case, the counselor acknowledged to the client the difficulty of utilizing condoms for some people, especially women, and that this was the image typically portrayed in the media. The client responded that she felt uncomfortable bringing the subject up, which correlates with her admission of the need to drink before engaging in sex. The counselor utilized verbal persuasion and some role-playing to increase the client's perception of self-efficacy. Suggestions and instructions were given about how to comfortably talk about sex. Examples were given concerning the use of a condom to extend the male's erection time, which could increase her pleasure, as well as how to make condom usage more pleasurable for the male. Messages were also provided to support her right to choose whether she wanted to engage in sexual contact. The counselor concluded the session by role-playing a scenario with the client about discussing condoms and insisting on their use in a sexual encounter.

CHAPTER 7

CASE THREE

This case is similar to Jill's so is examined in a cursory manner only. Mary (not her real name) also is a heterosexual female, age 22, who presented herself for testing with unprotected vaginal intercourse as her only risk. After reviewing her risk and background materials, the counselor turned to the RBD Scale (Table 7.4).

Mary displayed low perceptions of response efficacy with a total score of only 8. She scored moderate to high on her perceptions of self-efficacy (12). She displayed normal levels of perception of the seriousness of AIDS (15) and susceptibility (9) for her cohort. Her final discriminating value score was -4 [(8 response efficacy + 12 self-efficacy = 20 efficacy) - (15 severity + 9 susceptibility = 24 threat) = -4], indicating she is engaging in fear control processes. With this information, the counselor knew he would have to emphasize efficacy issues and avoid mention of severity and susceptibility issues. The counselor began by probing the client on the individual constructs.

Counselor: I see that you are unsure about whether or not condoms work in preventing HIV infection.

Mary: I really don't think they work, although I know some people say they do. I just read in [conservative religious magazine] about how terrible condoms are for protecting yourself. They talked about all kinds of studies that showed the virus can get through the condom. They gave all kinds of examples of women who had gotten HIV even when using condoms. So yeah, I don't think they work.

Table 7.4   Case Three (Mary)

For each of the following statements, please indicate how much you agree or disagree by circling the appropriate response on a scale of 1 to 5, where "1" means "strongly disagree" and "5" means "strongly agree."

	Strongly Disagree			Strongly Agree
1. Using condoms is effective in preventing AIDS.	1	(2)	3	4	5
2. Condoms work in preventing AIDS.	1	(2)	3	4	5 ΣRE = 8
3. If I use a condom, I am less likely to get AIDS.	1	2	3	(4)	5
4. Using condoms to prevent AIDS is convenient.	1	2	3	(4)	5
5. Using condoms to prevent AIDS is easy.	1	2	3	4	(5) ΣSE = 12
6. I am able to use condoms to prevent getting AIDS.	1	2	(3)	4	5
					ΣEFFICACY = 20
7. I believe that AIDS is severe.	1	2	3	4	(5)
8. I believe that AIDS is a significant disease.	1	2	3	4	(5) ΣSEV = 15
9. I believe that AIDS is serious.	1	2	3	4	(5)
10. It is likely that I will contract AIDS.	1	2	(3)	4	5
11. I am at risk for getting AIDS.	1	2	(3)	4	5 ΣSUSC = 9
12. It is possible that I will contract AIDS.	1	2	(3)	4	5
					ΣTHREAT = 24
			DISCRIMINATING VALUE		−4

Counselor:	Have you ever used condoms?
Mary:	Yeah, I've used them but I don't like them. It's always so uncomfortable to bring them up. It's like, you're really getting romantic, the mood is great, and then you have to stop, dig out a condom, open it up, put in on, and by that time you've killed the mood. Besides, if they don't work anyway, then why use them?

Based on these statements, it was clear the counselor needed to refute Mary's response efficacy beliefs, which apparently were generated by an article on the unreliability of condoms appearing in a conservative religious magazine. In addition, the counselor needed to role-play how to use condoms without breaking the mood to increase Mary's perceptions of self-efficacy. Next, the counselor asked questions about the threat dimensions.

Counselor:	I see that you think AIDS is a severe disease.
Mary:	Yes.
Counselor:	And you think you're somewhat susceptible to getting it?
Mary:	Not any more.
Counselor:	What? Why not?
Mary:	Because I'm not having sex anymore. I've decided to become celibate until I marry—when and if I ever marry.

This response greatly surprised the counselor given Mary's previous sexual activity level. We could assume that her decision is an example of a danger control response because becoming celibate would presumably eliminate the danger. The problem is that celibacy is not Mary's desired normal state, according to her precounseling survey. In addition, according to human sexuality research, this decision may be a maladaptive response to extreme fear. In most health education courses, professionals are taught to promote positive, healthy ways of living as well as teach avoidance of negative behavioral patterns. If viewed through the lens of healthy human sexuality, Mary's decision to be celibate appears to be a fear control response and not conducive to her well-being.

The messages developed for Mary avoided any references to the severity of AIDS or to her potential susceptibility to AIDS. They focused exclusively on response and self-efficacy issues. Respected, contemporary reports and studies were shown to demonstrate the efficacy of condoms. However, great care was taken to only use materials the client would deem accurate (e.g., medical journals were seen as accurate; however, a liberal magazine like *Cosmopolitan*, was not). In addition, condoms were demonstrated for their strength and durability and resistance to leakage (filling up with water similar to a water balloon). Additional sexual activities (nonintercourse activities) that could be options for a healthy expression of sexuality were outlined. Messages were also given concerning the satisfaction and fulfillment realized from a positive perception of sexuality. Finally, the counselor role-played a romantic scenario with her, illustrating how the use of condoms could become part of, and not an interruption to, foreplay.

CHAPTER 7

CASE FOUR

Mark (not his real name) was a 21-year-old male who identified himself as gay and presented for counseling with unprotected oral intercourse, no ejaculation, as his only risk. This was his second counseling and testing appointment. After reviewing the client's risk and background assessments, the counselor turned to Mark's RBD Scale (Table 7.5).

Mark scored 14 out of a possible 15 on the items measuring response efficacy. This indicates that he strongly agrees that using condoms is an effective response. He scored 15 out of a possible 15 on the self-efficacy questions, which indicates that his perceptions of his ability to use condoms are also very strong. Further, his strong efficacy perceptions were also exhibited when he explained his rationale for being tested.

> **Counselor:** I see you are a strong believer in condoms and their use.
>
> **Mark:** When and if I engage in any form of anal and/or oral sex, I use them—no problem! I'm always very careful. Just to be sure, I get tested every six months.

Scored responses for severity of threat were normal for Mark's cohort (15). Counselors at this campus health center have found that gay clients almost never score below a perfect 15 on the severity of threat part of the scale. Mark's responses to the items measur-

Table 7.5   Case Four (Mark)

For each of the following statements, please indicate how much you agree or disagree by circling the appropriate response on a scale of 1 to 5, where "1" means "strongly disagree" and "5" means "strongly agree."

	Strongly Disagree				Strongly Agree
1. Using condoms is effective in preventing AIDS.	1	2	3	4	(5)
2. Condoms work in preventing AIDS.	1	2	3	(4)	5 ΣRE = 14
3. If I use a condom, I am less likely to get AIDS.	1	2	3	4	5
4. Using condoms to prevent AIDS is convenient.	1	2	3	4	(5)
5. Using condoms to prevent AIDS is easy.	1	2	3	4	(5) ΣSE = 15
6. I am able to use condoms to prevent getting AIDS.	1	2	3	4	(5)
					ΣEFFICACY = 29
7. I believe that AIDS is severe.	1	2	3	4	(5)
8. I believe that AIDS is a significant disease.	1	2	3	4	(5) ΣSEV = 15
9. I believe that AIDS is serious.	1	2	3	4	(5)
10. It is likely that I will contract AIDS.	(1)	2	3	4	5
11. I am at risk for getting AIDS.	1	2	(3)	4	5 ΣSUSC = 7
12. It is possible that I will contract AIDS.	1	2	(3)	4	5
					ΣTHREAT = 22
			DISCRIMINATING VALUE		+7

ing susceptibility to threat (7) were a little lower than normal for his cohort. One very low response appeared for the question concerning the likelihood that the client will contract AIDS. To this question, Mark responded "1" (Strongly Disagree). The client's final discriminating value was +7 [(14 response efficacy + 15 self-efficacy = 29 efficacy) - (15 severity + 7 susceptibility = 22 threat) = +7], indicating he is engaging in danger control responses. Message development and delivery centered on reinforcing and validating perceptions of response and self-efficacy, and questioning and increasing perceived susceptibility.

The earlier exchange showed that the client needed very little reinforcement on response and self-efficacy. Mark exhibited a confident manner concerning his sexual practices and the counselor was convinced that he did as he said. The counselor was perplexed by the low score on the susceptibility measure and probed this issue.

Counselor: I see you strongly disagree that there's any likelihood of you contracting AIDS.

Mark: I always use condoms. I always protect myself. I really believe that I won't get HIV because I play it safe.

Counselor: Well, do you know that people with your demographic profile who engage in the types of sexual behaviors you do are at highest risk for getting infected with HIV? It's really important that you understand this.

Mark: Look, I know all of the facts and figures, and I know how to protect myself, so I do. I really believe I'm doing a good job.

Counselor: Well, I would have to agree with you based on what you're saying. You're doing the right thing, using a condom anytime you have intercourse. I'm also glad to see you're committed to periodic HIV testing. I think you're doing a good job.

Because the counselor believed the client was doing everything he could to control the risk of HIV infection, he did not give additional threat messages and merely reinforced the client's current safe sex behaviors.

CONCLUSION ▪▪

This chapter illustrates the use of the Risk Behavior Diagnosis Scale in an HIV Counseling, Testing, and Referral site on a university campus. The threat utilized in this version of the scale was HIV and the response was condom use. The scale was administered to clients who presented themselves for HIV counseling and testing. This chapter showed how the scale could numerically discriminate between individuals who were engaging in fear control and danger control processes, and help counselors develop effective and targeted health risk messages. Remember, this chapter shows just one application of the RBD Scale. Any kind of health threat and recommended response can be inserted into the scale. Indeed, the scale has been used in nutrition counseling, a hearing protection project, and a program to prevent beryllium disease, as well as in other situations.

CHAPTER 7

☷ NOTE

1. For purposes of this book, RBD Scales for the case studies appear with the scoring apparatus apparent, with spaces placed between the efficacy scale (questions 1 to 6) and the threat scale (questions 7 to 12), and with clear demarcations between response/self-efficacy and severity/susceptibility.

8

Data Collection

The next two chapters focus on data collection and analysis techniques. In these chapters, we introduce a number of ways to gather information and make sense of it. It is our position that the best health communication campaigns are developed and implemented by incorporating methods of data collection and analysis to assess the effects of your messages. Of course, the complexity of your methods depend on both your knowledge level and the needs of your campaign. The benefits obtained from some basic research on your campaign far outweigh the effort required, and provide the best chance of developing and implementing a successful health communication project. Once you have become familiar with the basic techniques of data collection and analysis, you can use them repeatedly in all of your health communication projects. After working through the next two chapters, you should be able to collect and analyze data yourself, as well as read reports and studies related to your topic conducted by other health communication professionals.

TYPES OF EVALUATION ▓

Before exploring data collection and analysis techniques, let's spend some time differentiating among the most common types of evaluation. In Chapter 5, you were introduced to formative evaluation. In addition, we discuss in this chaper process evaluation and outcome evaluation. Even though the purpose of each type of evaluation differs, the techniques of data collection and analysis can be used in all of them.

Formative Evaluation

Formative evaluation may be defined as the "systematic incorporation of feedback about one or more components of a planned activity before communication with a target audience" (Meyer & Dearing, 1996, p.46). Quite simply, formative evaluation gives you an opportunity to learn about your target audience and their preferences before you *develop and implement* your health communication program. As noted in Chapter 5, formative evaluation can be used to learn about your target audience's perceptions toward the health risk and recommended responses, as well as their preferences for receiving messages from various sources and channels. The type of formative evaluation referred to in Chapter 5 is preproduction research because the information is collected before any messages or other program materials are developed (Atkin & Freimuth, 1989). However, another important aspect of formative evaluation is postproduction research, which is used to gather perceptions from target audience members about program messages or materials that have been produced, but not yet "introduced" to target audience members (e.g., pamphlets, posters, public service announcements, videos, etc.). So, preproduction formative evaluation is conducted to help you develop relevant, useful, and appropriate materials, and postproduction formative evaluation ensures you "got it right." Whether you engage in one or both types of formative evaluation, the time and money spent is well worth the effort. And although formative evaluation cannot guarantee program success, it helps you identify and correct potentially costly shortcomings as well as relatively minor deficiencies, thereby increasing the likelihood of success. As we said in Chapter 5, *up-front work saves tail-end work.*

Process Evaluation

Process evaluation is conducted after your program has begun but before it ends, perhaps even several times during the program. A process evaluation helps determine whether your program is being conducted as intended, relative to expectations established prior to the beginning of the campaign. Questions asked in a process evaluation commonly focus on the activities performed; their frequency, location, and time; persons served by the activities; and finally, how they were performed (Meyer, 1997).

This information is important for several reasons. First, it enables you to make changes if you find some aspects of your program are not enacted according to plan. For example, imagine you have developed a public service announcement and made arrangements with a particular television station to show it three times each day for six weeks. After two weeks, you find that your PSA was not shown at all during the first week, and only nine times the second week. At this point, you may choose to contact the television station to determine why your PSA has not been shown as agreed, and to make arrangements to correct the problem.

To further exemplify how a process evaluation can lead to programmatic changes, consider the following case study concerning the conduct of a bar outreach program focusing on HIV prevention. Program coordinators stuffed large envelopes with several brochures, a condom, and a tube of lubricant. After distributing these envelopes at a bar, they noticed something interesting over the next several evenings—namely that the wastebaskets at the bar were full of their large envelopes. Thinking that the patrons simply didn't want them, they decided to reuse those that were not soiled. To their surprise, some of the envelopes were empty, but most contained only the brochures. Patrons took the condom, lubricant, and perhaps one brochure, stuffed these items in a pocket or purse, and discarded the unwanted envelope. From this assessment, health educators realized that the contents were not the problem as much as the method used for distribution. Shortly thereafter, they developed a "safe sex kit" approximately the size of a credit card although a bit thicker. They managed to include all of the same information on small targeted cards (rather than brochures) and replaced the tube of lubricant with a flat container (no change was necessary for the condom). Now, patrons who received the "safe sex kit" could easily and discretely place it in a pocket or purse for later reference or use. An examination of wastebaskets revealed that campaign materials were no longer being thrown away.

In addition to the ability to make changes in your program, sometimes it is important simply to document the fact that all program activities were conducted as intended. The reason is that you often cannot say your program resulted in the desired effect unless you can substantiate it was carried out as planned.

To illustrate, consider the following example based on an actual process evaluation conducted by one of the authors. The program was a school-based curriculum designed to reduce violence among teenagers. It consisted of 12 lessons to be taught using specific materials. If behaviors among the teens changed after the curriculum, then it could be concluded the curriculum was effective. To confirm this, however, first substantiation that the lessons were, in fact, taught as intended was needed. To be sure, a research assistant randomly visited the classrooms of all four teachers in the schools using the curriculum to verify the lessons were being taught appropriately. This process evaluation revealed that teachers were all presenting the curriculum as directed.

Information for a process evaluation may be obtained directly from target audience members, from individuals providing the messages (e.g., health educators, teachers, television stations), or sometimes through direct observation, as in the previous example. As with formative evaluation, we strongly recommend you conduct some type of process evaluation, and we assure you that the rewards relative to the effort are substantial.

Outcome or Summative Evaluation

The third and final type of evaluation discussed here is outcome evaluation, undertaken to answer the question, "what effect did my health communication program have on target audience members?" This evaluation is most typically conducted after the health communication program has been completed, although additional outcome evaluations may be conducted during the program especially if it has distinct phases. Often the desired effect is some type of behavior change (e.g., smoking cessation, condom use, or regular exercise), although sometimes the objective is to change the knowledge, attitudes, or beliefs of target audience members. Although this may seem relatively straightforward, determining your program's effect on target audience members can be quite challenging. Nonetheless, an outcome evaluation may be the most beneficial type of evaluation you conduct. After all, do you want to continue investing valuable time and money on a health communication program that doesn't produce the desired outcomes, or worse, has the opposite effect, on your target audience? Of course, if you follow our advice and conduct both formative and process evaluation, it is likely your program will have the desired effect. But you never know for sure unless you also conduct an outcome evaluation.

So, how do you conduct an outcome evaluation? Unfortunately, there is no simple or consistent answer to this question. It really depends on the amount of time, money, and expertise you allocate to the evaluation. We discuss three different designs for outcome evaluation, along with their strengths and weaknesses. Ultimately, you must decide which one best suits your programmatic needs. The designs we focus on include (a) the posttest-only design, (b) the pretest/posttest design, and (c) the pretest/posttest control group design.

CHAPTER 8

Posttest-only Design

One of the easiest and most commonly used methods is called a posttest-only design. Here, information is collected from target audience members only after they are exposed to the health risk messages. This design should sound familiar to you because it is the method almost always used to assign course grades at all levels of education. Think about it. You walked into class, were exposed to certain messages (i.e., the curriculum), and then were tested to determine what you knew. This evaluation method is advantageous in that it is relatively fast, easy, and inexpensive to conduct and analyze. But have you ever stopped to consider the validity of this procedure? If you are similar to most people, the answer is "no."

We make the assumption that if people can answer a certain number or percentage of questions correctly, then the program (class) as well as the individuals are a success. But are they? How do you know, for example, that the messages didn't confuse them, and that perhaps without the course, they would have answered even more questions correctly? Additionally, how can you be sure that the demonstrated knowledge came from the class and not from other sources such as the Internet or television programs? The answer is you really cannot be certain with a posttest-only design.

The same dilemma exists for health communicators. How can you be sure that your program, designed to increase the use of bicycle helmets, for example, worked, when all you know is how many people wore them after exposure to your messages? The answer is, you don't. You don't know if people wore helmets more after your program, before your program, or if they wore them just as much as before. Nor do you know whether your specific messages influenced them. Perhaps something completely unrelated to your messages persuaded individuals to wear the helmets. For example, perhaps a famous person was severely injured in a bicycle accident and began to advocate the use of helmets. What caused your target audience to wear helmets? The famous person's messages or your campaign? However, although a posttest-only design is a relatively weak design, it's better than nothing. If a posttest-only evaluation is the only one you can afford, then you can strengthen the link between your campaign and its effects by asking questions such as,

- What caused you to wear your helmet?
- Have you heard any messages promoting helmet use recently?
- If yes, what were those messages?

In other words, try to assess whether your campaign messages are related to people's actions.

Pretest/Posttest Design

In the pretest/posttest design of outcome evaluation, information is collected both before and after your health risk messages have been disseminated. The idea behind this design is to determine the knowledge, attitudes, beliefs, and/or behaviors of target audience members up front, before they are exposed to your messages. After your health communication program, you make the same assessment (typically using the same instrument). The primary advantage of this design is that the extent of change among audience members can be gauged. You can determine, for example, whether a greater number of target audience members use condoms, exercise regularly, or wear bicycle safety helmets, than did prior to your campaign. Although the addition of a pretest provides information about changes in your target audience, it cannot assure that the observed changes are actually the result of your effort, your program, or your messages. After all, it is still possible that people changed because of some other health program or well-publicized event that moved them to act. Again, the pretest/posttest design is better than nothing and significantly improves on the posttest-only design. But, you cannot directly connect target audience members' changes in behavior to your campaign or something that happened during your campaign. However, from a pragmatic viewpoint, do what is best given your resources and skills and use this design if you can link your campaign messages to behavioral effects.

Pretest/Posttest with Control Group Design

This third outcome evaluation design addresses the problem of determining whether your program is responsible for observed changes and is the strongest design presented here. The pretest/ posttest with control group design is similar to the pretest/ posttest design in that observations are made both before and after the health program is administered. The addition of the control group means that the pretest and posttest are administered to groups of individuals who are either exposed to your health risk messages (your target audience) or not (the control group).

There are two types of control groups you can consider. With a true control group, you can *randomly assign* members of your target audience into the experimental group or control group. Note that *random assignment* is different from *random selection*, where individuals are randomly selected from a defined population. Probability theory suggests that by randomly assigning individuals into (at least) two different groups, any pre-intervention differences among people should be evenly distributed across your experimental and control groups. Therefore, idiosyncrasies in your target audience members should be equally represented in both the experimental and control groups. As a result, your outcome should be influenced by your intervention only, and not by some preexisting characteristics of your target audience.

For example, say you were running a physical fitness campaign at a high school. You would want to make sure all individuals across campus—athletes as well as non-athletes—were evenly represented in both your intervention and control group. If you simply gave your intervention to some campus clubs and not others, then you run the risk that the unique characteristics of each club might influence the outcome and not your intervention. For instance, say all the athletic clubs fell into the control group and the non-athletic clubs fell into the intervention group. You might find no difference at the end of your campaign—not because your campaign failed, but because the control group was already physically fit and, therefore, did not have as much room to shift as the other group. Fortunately, randomizing by individuals prevents this problem because each group would have some athletes and some non-athletes. Using a true control group, to which members of your target audience have been randomly assigned, as they have to the intervention group, is the best design you can use because you can be relatively sure any changes in the intervention group result from your intervention alone, and not some other factor.

To randomize members of your target audience into two or more groups, you simply take a group of people and place some into the intervention group and some into the control group via a randomization procedure. You can use a random numbers table (found in the back of most statistics books), or more easily, simply put everyone's name on a piece of paper, shuffle them together in a hat or bag, and then draw names. For instance, the first name drawn goes into the experimental group, the second name drawn goes into the control group, the third name drawn goes into the experimental group, and so on. If you can successfully randomize members of your target audience into experimental and control groups, then you're on your way to a rigorous and thorough test of your intervention. However, there's one more issue you need to be aware of to make sure that any differences in behaviors following the intervention result from the intervention alone—contamination of conditions.

Say you gathered all of the high school students' names at All-Star High School into a paper bag, and then you randomly drew names to make up your intervention and control groups. The principal even agreed to have a special assembly just for your intervention while the students in the control group got an extra long lunch period (no intervention). You've done everything right to this point. But, suppose now that the students attending the intervention assembly tell those students who were at the extended lunch all about the assembly. Your control group has just been contaminated. That is, it has been exposed to at least part of your intervention and you no longer can have a clean test between groups of your intervention.

To avoid contamination of conditions, you must make sure that members of your target audience do not talk to members of your control group about the intervention. This might be difficult to do with students but is probably easier to do with adult audiences who may not even know each other in the first place. We've had great success administering "clean" interventions (i.e., where those in the intervention group don't talk about the intervention to those in the control group) just by asking members of each group not to talk to each other for a certain time period (e.g., one month). We appeal to study participants' altruism by making them feel part of an important research project and emphasizing that all our efforts would be in vain if members of other groups talked with each other about the study. Of course, if members of your study groups don't know each other, then contamination of conditions is even less of a problem.

The other type of control group is technically called a "comparison" group. In these situations, the researcher uses already intact groups and simply assigns one group to receive the intervention and the other to act as a comparison group. While this practice is far less preferred than the randomly assigned control group because of the potential of pre-intervention differences (as in the high school student example above), it sometimes is the only realistic method available. And, an evaluation with a comparison group is much stronger and more rigorous than an evaluation that looks at only pre-intervention versus post-intervention differences. When using a comparison group as a control group, take great care to match as many characteristics as possible between the two groups to ensure the test of your intervention is sound. In the case of the high school student example, because of the significant pre-intervention differences on the topic of your intervention (physical fitness), you probably should use the non-athletes (because there's more room for change on physical fitness measures) and find a comparison group at another, similar school with a similar group of non-athletes. By doing this, the test of your intervention would be fairer and more revealing.

Table 8.1 summarizes each evaluation type discussed thus far in terms of its purpose, stage of the campaign, data collection methods, and cost.

▪▪ GATHERING DATA FOR THE EVALUATION

Now that you are familiar with three different evaluation methods, we turn to data collection, or the process of gathering information. As we suggested earlier, no single

Table 8.1 Types of Evaluation

	Formative	*Process*	*Outcome*
Purpose	To inform campaign decisions about target audience, activities, materials, delivery methods, etc.	To document that the activities were conducted and done so in an appropriate manner	To ascertain the effect of the campaign on target audience members
Stage of Campaign	Conducted prior to the start of the campaign	Conducted during the campaign	Conducted after the campaign, or after a part of it has concluded
Common Methods	Interviews, focus groups, surveys	Interviews, observations, written records	Surveys, written records
Cost	Low to moderate	Low	Moderate to high

method of data collection should be used to conduct a formative, process, or outcome evaluation. Any of the techniques described here could be applied to any type of evaluation. The data collection method(s) you ultimately select depend on a number of factors including the time, money, and expertise you can allocate to the evaluation.

We first discuss three ways to collect data from individuals including (a) in-person interviews, (b) telephone interviews, and (c) mailed questionnaires, and then move to group data collection, specifically, the focus group interview. After that, we discuss questionnaire development and end the chapter with a brief discussion of sampling procedures.

DATA COLLECTION METHODS ▪▪

Several different ways for collecting data from individuals exist, each with specific strengths and weaknesses (see Table 8.2). The in-person interview is conducted with the interviewer (i.e., health educator) and the interviewee (e.g., target audience member[s]) physically located in the same place. An important distinction exists between such an in-person interview and an in-person, self-administered survey. In the first case, the interviewer typically reads questions to a single interviewee and records the answers as they are given. One advantage of this method is that the interviewer has a great deal of control over the interview and can ensure that the interviewee is focused on the questions being asked. Perhaps more important, the interviewer can more easily determine if the interviewee is confused by assessing nonverbal as well as verbal cues, and is immediately available to answer questions. In-person interviews do have some limitations, however. Most notably, they are relatively more expensive to conduct. The cost in terms of the interviewer's time increases substantially if s/he is required to go to multiple locations (e.g., individual's homes, places of work, clinics, etc.) to conduct the interviews.

When an in-person, self-administered survey is conducted, a written questionnaire is typically distributed to many, sometimes even hundreds, of interviewees. The interviewer clearly loses some control over the process with so many respondents, but the interviewer is still present to administer the survey and answer any questions. The greatest advantage of the in-person, self-administered survey is that a large amount of data can be collected in a relatively short period of time.

Table 8.2 Methods of Data Collection

	In-Person, Self-Administered Survey	In-Person Interview	Telephone Interview	Mailed, Self-Administered Survey
Cost	Low	High	Moderate	Low-moderate
Data Quality				
Response rate	High	High	Moderate	Low
Respondent motivation	Moderate	High	Moderate	Low
Interviewer bias	Low	Moderate-high	Low	None-low
Ability to clarify and probe	Low	High	High	None
Ability to use visual aids	Moderate-high	High	None	Low-moderate
Speed	High	Low	Moderate	Low-moderate
Anonymity	Moderate-high	Low	Moderate-high	High
Control of context and question order	Low	High	High	None-low

A second way to gather information is through telephone interviews. The telephone interview offers some of the same advantages as the in-person interview, the most important being the opportunity to clarify any questions the interviewee might have at the time of the interview. The primary difference, however, is that the interviewer cannot assess nonverbal cues, and therefore must rely more on the interviewee to verbalize any confusion. The telephone survey may also be less expensive than the face-to-face interview. The telephone interview may be conducted virtually anywhere the interviewer can find a telephone and is thus, much more convenient as well. Of course, cellular telephones offer the interviewer more flexibility today than in the past. The primary disadvantage of conducting telephone interviews is that the interviewee may not be available when the interviewer calls. In fact, it is not uncommon for the interviewer to call three or more times before speaking with the interviewee, to say nothing of the interviewee's availability when finally reached. One way to partially alleviate this difficulty is to contact interviewees in advance to schedule a convenient date and time to conduct the interview. Additionally, compared with the face-to-face interview, the likelihood of interruptions occurring is greater with a telephone interview.

A third way to collect information is through a mail survey. As its name suggests, questionnaires are mailed to respondents who are typically asked to complete them and mail them back to the interviewer. This method's advantages include its relatively lower costs and greater convenience for both the interviewer and the interviewee. After the interviewer assembles and mails the questionnaire, s/he simply waits for respondents to return them. It is recommended, however, that the interviewer send a follow-up letter or postcard to remind interviewees to complete and return the questionnaire. Mailed questionnaires are convenient for interviewees because they can complete the surveys whenever they desire.

As you might expect, though, this method also has its drawbacks. Perhaps most important, the response rate, that is, the number of surveys completed, is almost certainly lower compared with face-to-face or telephone interviews. It is easier for the potential respondent to dismiss the interview simply by throwing the questionnaire away. Even if the interviewee intends to complete the questionnaire at a later date, it can easily be put aside, forgotten, or even lost. Additionally, there is typically no opportunity for the interviewee to ask questions of or seek clarification from the interviewer, should this be necessary. Finally, the interviewer has no way to control for distractions or interruptions (e.g., television, telephone calls, etc.) that may occur while the respondent is completing the questionnaire.

Although individual interviews may be the most common way to collect information from respondents, situations may arise where it is advantageous to collect information from groups of people. The term, "groups of people" should not imply a roomful of individuals completing the questionnaire on their own. Rather, we refer here to a group-based interview in which individuals respond to questions collectively. The most common group interview is the focus group, which typically includes 6 to 9 participants. A focus group may be defined as "a carefully planned discussion designed to obtain perceptions on a defined area of interest in a permissive, non-threatening environment" (Krueger, 1988, p.18). Unlike individual interviews, the focus group interview emphasizes interaction among interviewees and thereby enables respondents to feed off each other's responses. The small number of participants used in a focus group gives each member sufficient opportunity to contribute to the discussion without isolating any one person and usually elicits a diversity of perspectives. Individuals, in fact, are encouraged to disagree with others in the focus group, as the idea is not to determine a definitive, "correct" answer to a question, but rather to elicit a variety of opinions based on individual perceptions. In addition to enabling respondents to feed off each other, focus groups are advantageous in that the information obtained is relatively rich and detailed, the interviewer may probe into certain topics not previously examined (based on the discussion), and the information is relatively less expensive to obtain, at least compared with asking the same questions of 6 to 9 respondents individually.

Focus groups do have some drawbacks, however. First, a trained individual, referred to as the moderator, must keep the discussion focused, ensure all respondents contribute, and be familiar enough with the topic to ensure appropriate information is being collected. With this background, it should be evident why focus groups are especially useful in the postproduction, formative stage of program design. It enables the health educator to collect a diversity of opinions and reactions to messages developed but not yet disseminated to target audience members.

Questionnaire Development

No matter how you decide to collect the data, you need to develop one or more interview protocols. An interview protocol consists of the topics and subtopics the interviewer discusses with respondents. The interview protocol also often includes the specific questions the interviewer asks. Some interviews are conducted by following the protocol precisely, that is, by asking the questions verbatim, without deviation or unintended probing. This is a highly structured interview, advantageous in that precisely the same information is collected from all respondents. As such, the interview is easier to conduct and the results relatively easier to analyze. Of course, if the information is

CHAPTER 8

not collected in-person or by telephone, it is difficult to ensure the questions are answered in the precise order desired.

The unstructured interview differs markedly from the structured interview. Here, the protocol typically contains only a list of topics and perhaps, some subtopics to be covered. The interviewer is free to cover the topics in any order desired, and is also encouraged to probe, that is, to dig deeper into any topic, if so desired. The unstructured interview is advantageous in that it gives the interviewer a great deal of flexibility depending on how the interview unfolds. As you might suspect however, an unstructured interview is more difficult to conduct and the associated results more difficult to analyze. Perhaps the most common approach is to conduct a moderately structured interview, where the questions and order are determined ahead of time, but where the interviewer has the freedom to deviate from this discussion guide should the need arise. This approach is used often because it provides the interviewer with a high degree of both structure and flexibility.

Developing Interview Questions

Because most interviews are conducted with a moderate or high degree of structure, we turn our attention to the process of developing questions for the interview protocol. One of the most important factors the interviewer must consider is whether to use open-ended questions, closed-ended questions, or a combination of the two. Open-ended questions provide the interviewee with a great deal of latitude in response (Stewart & Cash, 2000). If you ever answered an essay question on an examination, then chances are you have answered an open-ended question. Some examples of open-ended questions a health educator might ask are

- How do you feel about wearing a bicycle safety helmet?
- What do you think you can do to prevent the spread of HIV?
- Do you think you are susceptible to skin cancer? Why or why not?

As you can see, the interviewee answering each of these questions can decide the length and type of information to provide. In general, open-ended questions are not perceived as threatening by interviewees, because they can respond as they see fit. Perhaps the biggest advantage of open-ended questions, however, is they elicit information as to *why* interviewees feel a certain way. That is, open-ended questions provide very rich, in-depth information. An open-ended question, for example, enables the health educator to find out why respondents engage in risky sexual behaviors, along with the fact that they do. The primary disadvantage of using open-ended questions is that responses can be quite time-consuming, and as such, the interviewer is limited in terms of how many topics can be covered and how many questions can be asked. Additionally, responses to open-ended questions are relatively more difficult and time-consuming to analyze, requiring a greater level of expertise. Finally, many respondents do not like to take the time to write out their responses. Therefore, it is often up to the interviewer to accurately capture the responses of the interviewee.

Closed-ended questions, on the other hand, restrict responses by suggesting, either explicitly or implicitly, how the interviewee should answer the question. Think again about examinations you have taken in the past. Multiple choice and true/false questions are examples of closed-ended questions as are various types of scaled questions. In the latter case, the respondent is asked, for example, to indicate the extent of agreement with a statement and provided with a scale ranging from "strongly agree" to "strongly disagree." Health educators may ask a multiple choice question such as, "Which of the following sources do you most trust to provide accurate health risk messages about AIDS?" and then provide a list of sources from which to select (e.g., the Surgeon General, the Centers for Disease Control and Prevention, state health department, or local AIDS prevention organization). To determine interviewees' susceptibility to bicycle injuries, the interviewer may simply ask "Do you believe you could be involved in a bicycle accident?" The implicitly suggested response is either "yes" or "no."

Notice the difference in the type of information obtained from these closed-ended questions. Respondents may indicate, for example, they trust the CDC the most, they do not feel susceptible to bicycle injuries, and they strongly agree with the statement, "Condoms effectively prevent the spread of HIV." However, the interviewer does not know *why* the respondents feel the way they do. While this is probably the major shortcoming of closed-ended questions, they do offer several advantages. Closed-ended questions can be answered fairly quickly and as a result, more topics and many more questions can be covered. In additional, closed-ended questions take little effort to complete on the part of the respondent and are relatively easier to analyze.

Most interview protocols contain a combination of open-ended and closed-ended questions. By including both, the interviewer can ascertain not only what respondents think or feel, but also why they think or feel a certain way. Of course, fewer topics can be covered when open-ended questions are included. However, in all likelihood, the benefits obtained from ascertaining in-depth information outweigh the costs. In reality, the decision to use only open-ended questions, only closed-ended questions, or some combination of the two depends on the purpose for collecting the information in the first place. Relatively more open-ended questions may be used, for example, when conducting a formative evaluation, but relatively more closed-ended questions may be more appropriate in an outcome evaluation.

RELIABILITY AND VALIDITY ■■

Two issues to consider in data collection are the validity and reliability of the questions. A question is valid when it measures what you suggest it measures. To put it another way, validity concerns whether your question actually measures or "gets at" the concept you are interested in measuring (e.g., susceptibility to HIV). Reliability, on the other hand, refers to the consistency of your questions or measurements. One aspect of reliability, external reliability, focuses on the extent to which you would obtain the same results if you asked the question or took the measurement more than once.

Think about the pretest/posttest design discussed earlier in this chapter. Your questions are reliable if respondents answered in a similar fashion both times. Internal reliability focuses on a different type of consistency, namely the extent to which all questions associated with a particular concept contribute equally to the results. This is an important consideration if you ask respondents multiple questions about a topic.

An easy way to remember the concepts of validity and reliability is the example of weighing yourself. Imagine that you step on a scale today to see how much you weigh. Because scales are designed to measure how much an object weighs, we say the scale is a valid measure of your weight. That is, the scale measures what it is supposed to measure. But say you wanted to assess your intelligence level with the scale. Would the scale then be a valid measure? Of course not. To measure intelligence, you would likely use one of the various tests designed to measure intelligence. Now, let's consider reliability. Imagine that you weigh yourself on the same scale each day for a week and each time you do so, the weight is approximately the same, making allowances for slight differences resulting from variations in eating or exercise habits, for example. In this case, we say the scale (measure) is both valid (it measures what it is supposed to) and reliable (consistent results are obtained upon repeated measurement). But what if you obtained drastically different results each time you weighed yourself, perhaps differing by as much as 25 pounds from day to day? In that case, we say the measure, that is, the scale, is valid, but not reliable because different results were obtained each time you weighed yourself. Ideally, of course, we want to use measures that are both valid and reliable.

▦ SAMPLE SIZE

One question often asked about data collection is "How many people should I collect data from?" Although this is a reasonable and seemingly straightforward question, the answer is anything but simple. Let's begin by thinking about the reason we collect information in the first place. We collect information to answer questions about our target audience, such as how susceptible do they believe they are to a particular threat (formative evaluation question) and to what extent behaviors changed as a result of the health risk messages (outcome evaluation question). Of course, if you want to know how your target audience feels or has changed, beyond any doubt, simply ask *everyone*, and you will know. The feasibility of collecting information from everyone, however, is rather low because most of us don't have the time, money, or will to do so. Imagine, for example, trying to collect information from a target audience comprised of all teens between the ages of 13 and 17 in the city of Los Angeles. Clearly, this would be an impossible task.

Fortunately, we can still have a very high level of confidence in our results without collecting data from every single person in the target audience. Still, the question as to the size of the sample persists. We now know the answer is somewhere between zero and "everyone," but how many? The answer depends on how strong an effect you expect from your campaign. If you are using the variables described in this book, the EPPM in particular, we know from past research that you can expect a moderately large effect size on attitudes, intentions, and behaviors from interventions that focus on threat and efficacy.[1] The degree of confidence desired in the results represents another component in determining the number of people from whom to collect data. The most commonly acceptable confidence level is 95%, which means that we want to be 95% certain our findings are not the result of chance or error. Although this is the regularly accepted confidence level, circumstances may dictate that you specify a higher level of confidence (e.g., when testing the effects of an experimental drug) or accept a lower confidence level (e.g., when exploring a topic not yet well studied). The important point to note is that the number of individuals you need to question increases, all else equal, as the desired level of confidence increases. That is, the more certain you want to be that your results are "real," the more people you need to collect data from. So, the two variables we need to consider to determine the appropriate number of people to include in data collection are the effect size you expect from your intervention and the level of confidence you want in your results.

Based on previous EPPM research, the following is a rule of thumb. For survey or interview research, where you're randomly selecting individuals from a target population, you need approximately 150 persons to assess relationships between variables. A survey or interview study with this many participants provides enough "power" to detect significant relationships between variables, if significant relationships exist. When you're comparing groups, as you would for an outcome evaluation (where you compare those exposed to your intervention with those in a control or comparison group), you need 30 to 40 people per group to detect significant differences between groups, if significant differences exist. These numbers err on the side of caution and represent the optimal number of participants needed. Of course, you could collect data from fewer people if you simply want to get an idea of people's perceptions and behaviors.

Once you know how many individuals are required, you may still wonder how to determine which individuals from whom to collect data. Typically, researchers choose a *random sample* from their target population to get a *representative* sample of the entire target audience, so they can *generalize* their results to this target audience. Random sampling is different from random assignment. Random sampling refers to the process of randomly selecting individuals from your population to whom you might ask questions. Random assignment, as discussed earlier, refers to the process of randomly assigning members of your target audience into either an intervention or control group. Random sampling ensures you have the best representation possible of your entire audience, with all of their idiosyncrasies and quirks. Therefore, *random sampling* is more concerned with external validity, also called generalizability, or the degree to which your study's results are valid and represent your entire population's tendencies or opinions. Random sampling is used most often in surveys and interviews where you're just trying to collect information on attitudes, perceptions, behaviors, and so on. In contrast, random assignment is most often used when comparing two or more groups to assess an intervention's effectiveness. *Random assignment* is more concerned with internal validity, or the degree to which your intervention's results are the result of your intervention alone and no other factors.

In terms of random sampling, ideally, you don't select anyone yourself, but rather rely on a process to select them for you. In fact, the sample size recommended in tables is based on the presumption that the actual sample drawn is done so in an unbiased manner.

The most common method used to enable you to draw an unbiased sample is called *simple random sampling*. This methods gives each individual in the population (target audience) an equal opportunity to be selected for inclusion in the study. Imagine you want to draw a simple random sample from all students at a particular university. One way to do this is to put everyone's name in a hat (probably a large hat) and select names until you have drawn the number of persons needed to make up your sample. Although there are many ways to draw a random sample, the point is that individuals are selected at random, and as such, they should well represent the target audience.

CHAPTER 8

SUMMARY ■■

In this chapter, we discussed the process of data collection. We began with a discussion of three types of evaluation that require data collection. Each type of evaluation—formative, process, and outcome—serves a different, but important purpose. You have the best chance for success by using each type of evaluation, although depth and sophistication vary, depending on your campaign. Regardless of the types of evaluation used or the sophistication level, you should give each type of evaluation careful thought before beginning the campaign. Waiting until the campaign is underway or finished to think about evaluation may compromise your ability to conduct the necessary evaluation.

We also reviewed several different methods of data collection in this chapter, each having its own strengths and weaknesses. Ultimately, the methods you decide to use depend on the type of evaluation you conduct and the specific information or data you hope to collect. Developing measurement tools to assess the effects of your campaign is an extremely important, yet often overlooked, activity. It takes much thought to develop a set of cohesive topics and associated questionnaire items that are both valid and reliable. In the end, however, the time spent is well worth it because you can then state with confidence the specific results of your campaign.

:: NOTE

1. Power analysis, or analysis to determine how many individuals are needed to detect differences if differences, in fact, exist between groups, is highly technical. A thorough discussion is beyond the scope of this book. We refer readers to J. Cohen (1988).

In six EPPM studies by Witte, effect sizes ranged from medium to very large, with an average effect size of $d = .77$ for attitudes, $d = .64$ for intentions, and $d = .80$ for behaviors. To meet conventional standards of .80 power with alpha = .05 (one-tailed tests), 29 persons per group are needed for attitudes, 38 persons are needed per group for intentions, and 26 persons are needed per group for behaviors. To test correlations, approximately 66 participants are needed to test the relationship between efficacy and attitudes, intentions, and behaviors; approximately 150 participants are needed to test the relationship between threat and attitudes, intentions, and behaviors.

9

Data Analysis

fter reading chapter 8 and completing the worksheets on data collection, you should feel reasonably confident in your ability to collect useful data for your evaluation. But what comes next? Now that you have worked hard to collect information, what do you do with it? If you are thinking data analysis, you are correct, and in this chapter we present some basic techniques of data analysis that enable you to make sense of the data and answer questions asked in the evaluation.

Although we discuss qualitative analysis in this chapter, the emphasis is on techniques of quantitative data analysis, and especially those methods you are most likely to use as a health educator/communicator. We focus on quantitative data analysis because, although most agencies are happy to hear anecdotes about the effectiveness of your intervention, in reality, most are not satisfied (i.e., willing to fund more projects) unless they have cold, hard numbers backing up the stories of success. Our goal is to demystify statistics and make it easy for you to offer numerical evidence to your funding sources. Specifically, we discuss frequency distributions, measures of central tendency and dispersion, and one test of difference between groups—the *t* test.

ANALYZING DATA

Analysis of data depends in large part on the questions you asked in the first place. Open-ended questions, such as, "What concerns do you have about your ability to enact the recommended behavior?" which give the respondent great flexibility in answering, are typically analyzed qualitatively. Closed-ended questions, on the other hand, such as, "Which of the following three barriers to enacting the recommended behavior concerns you the most?" provide the respondent with specific response categories (three in this case). These types of questions are usually analyzed quantitatively. Of course, if your questionnaire protocol included both open- and closed-ended questions, then you need to use both qualitative and quantitative procedures to analyze your data. First, let's take a brief look at qualitative analysis.

Qualitative Analysis

As its name suggests, a qualitative analysis considers the quality rather than the quantity of the responses. Unfortunately, there are no standardized methods for analyzing qualitative data as there are for analyzing quantitative data (Yin, 1988). Therefore, as you analyze your data, you may want to revisit the purpose of your interview, and let the problems direct your analysis (Krueger, 1988). Imagine, for example, you have finished conducting a focus group interview designed to ascertain respondents' perceptions of the threat (susceptibility and severity) of skin cancer and their corresponding efficacy levels (response and self-efficacy) to prevent its occurrence. In your focus group, it's likely you've asked one or more questions about each of these concepts. As such, you probably want to begin by analyzing each concept separately (i.e., analyze the responses about severity, susceptibility, response efficacy, and self-efficacy separately).

Before you start analyzing the data, you need to be sure you are very familiar with the data you have collected. The best way to do this is to review the notes you (or an assistant) took during the focus group (or interview). One way to be sure no important data are omitted is to use a tape recorder and record the interview. Using a tape recorder is advantageous because you can listen to the entire interview again or go back to a particularly important section any time you choose. It also allows you to review a section should you find your written notes are incomplete. However, even when you tape record an interview, you (or an assistant) should still take notes just in case there is a problem with the recorder. In any case, before you use a tape recorder, obtain permission from your respondents. We've found that most respondents don't mind the tape recorder if you explain its purpose. Furthermore, although there may be some concern respondents are affected by the tape recorder, we have found they usually forget about it after a few minutes and respond quite naturally.

To analyze the focus group (or interview—same procedures are used), you can either listen to the audiotape of the actual focus group and stop it whenever you need to write down key points, or have the audiotape professionally transcribed onto paper. It is much easier to work from a transcription than from the actual audiotape. While analyzing from an audiotape can be valuable because you get the general feel of a group as well as tone and strength of responses (e.g., mild versus strong), it also can be very time-consuming because you have to listen to a portion of the focus group, rewind it, listen again, and so on, until you understand what each person's points were. In contrast, when a typed transcription is in front of you, it's much easier to see the focus group as a whole, and link all discussions on a single topic or concept, even if they occurred at different times in the focus group or interview.

To analyze the focus groups, you first need to summarize what the group said about each of your key concepts. For example,

a. What did my focus group members say about the severity of skin cancer?
b. What did they say about their susceptibility to skin cancer?
c. What types of recommended responses did they suggest?
d. Did they think they could do these recommended responses?
e. Did they think the recommended responses would work to prevent skin cancer?

For many people, the analysis is complete after this step. They then simply report what the group said as a whole on each question or concept. Although no standardized method exists, your qualitative data analysis should be systematic. You should follow some procedure that allows others to understand exactly how you analyzed your data so that they can replicate it, if desired. For instance, in this example, you read transcriptions of the actual focus groups and then placed everyone's comments into one of five categories, letters "a" through "e" above. Another, more complicated analysis includes coding each person's responses according to your key concepts and then having someone else code the same transcripts for these responses. You then use a numerical formula to calculate inter-coder reliability. Many books on focus groups and interviews are available describing these more advanced procedures (e.g., Krueger, 1988; Sage series on methods and statistics, etc.). In general, health communicators can obtain a great deal of good information from the summary analysis described previously without the need to code the data, provided they clearly remove their biases and opinions from the research process by making sure that any information reported comes directly from the study participants and not from the researchers themselves.

Several points should be noted as you make sense of the qualitative data you have collected. First, you should always view the responses within the context of the question asked. Taking statements out of context can lead to faulty assumptions and conclusions that respondents never intimated. Additionally, you need to consider the actual words used by respondents and the way the words were stated (of course, this is easier to do when the interview has been recorded and transcribed). Even if the interview was not recorded, however, your notes should reflect specific words used and any important associated nonverbal communication. For example, an individual who feels "alarmed" by a particular threat feels different from an individual who feels "at risk" for the threat. Similarly, an individual who bangs the table with his hand while responding probably feels quite strongly about his response. By noting such specific strong words or actions, you can more accurately infer the meaning behind the specific response.

Finally, when reporting the results of your analysis, consider the distinction between reporting raw data, descriptive statements, and interpretive findings (Krueger, 1988). If you present raw data, you are providing exact quotes offered by respondents in the interview. Often, raw data are used when a specific quote perfectly illustrates a point you want to make. Descriptive statements differ from raw data in that you are not providing direct quotes, but rather descriptions or paraphrases of what one or more respondents said in the interview. To provide interpretive statements, you need to go beyond simple description or paraphrasing to make judgments or interpretations based on a synthesis of the information provided. This last method differs from the first two in that you, the analyst, give meaning to the information obtained in the interview. As stated previously, when interpreting the data, great care must be taken to truly reflect the interviewees without including any of your own opinions or biases.

Quantitative Analysis

Now let's turn to analyzing data quantitatively. As you might expect, the basis of a quantitative data analysis is in the quantification of the data collected. Quite simply, you are making sense of the data through numerical representation. Perhaps the easiest way to illustrate some of the techniques of quantitative data analysis is through examples.

Table 9.1 Frequency Table

Response Category	Number of Respondents Choosing This Answer
Strongly disagree	4
Disagree	2
Neutral/undecided	2
Agree	1
Strongly agree	1
Total	10

Frequencies

For ease of illustration, let's begin by looking at a single item (question) from your questionnaire designed to ascertain respondents' perceptions of their susceptibility to skin cancer. To determine an audience's level of perceived susceptibility, the following item was presented, "I am likely to develop skin cancer" and respondents were asked to indicate the extent to which they agreed or disagreed with this statement by selecting one of five responses:

I am likely to develop skin cancer.

1	2	3	4	5
Strongly Disagree	Disagree	Neutral	Agree	Strongly Agree

Let's assume your sample is comprised of 10 individuals whose responses to this item are illustrated in Table 9.1. The table is referred to as a frequency table and is typically the first tool you construct in most analyses. Table 9.1 depicts the frequency with which each response was selected, and furthermore, shows how the responses are distributed across response categories. Often, this information is presented in a bar graph, as in Figure 9.1.

A quick glance at Table 9.1 and Figure 9.1 reveals that many respondents do not feel susceptible to skin cancer, a few are undecided, and a few feel somewhat susceptible. This rudimentary analysis shows these respondents do not feel particularly susceptible to skin cancer as most of them answered "Neutral," "Disagree," or "Strongly Disagree." Although the information gleaned from the frequency distribution is useful, we can obtain more information by considering three measures of central tendency: (a) the mean, (b) the median, and (c) the mode.

Measures of Central Tendency

Measures of central tendency provide information about the clustering of responses within a distribution, which, in this case is your sample. By assuming an equal "distance" between response categories, we have assigned numerical values to each of the responses. That is, "Strongly Agree" equals "5;" "Agree" equals "4;" "Neutral" equals "3;" "Disagree" equals "2;" and "Strongly Disagree" equals "1." By assigning numbers, we know the higher the score, the more one feels susceptible to skin cancer, and the lower the score, the less susceptible one feels.

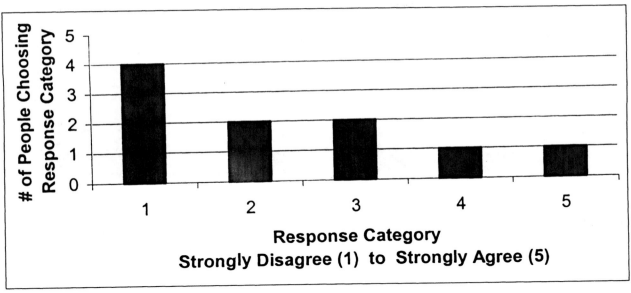

Figure 9.1 Bar Graph for Frequency Distribution

Now let's consider the first and most sensitive measure of central tendency, the *mean*. The mean score (technically the arithmetic mean) represents the average score obtained from all respondents. In school, your instructor may have indicated the mean score of an examination (although it was probably referred to as the "class average"). In baseball, the hitter's batting "average" is often computed and serves as an indication of productivity. Simply put, the mean score is computed by adding all scores in a distribution and dividing by the total number of scores. To compute the mean of an examination then, all scores would be added together and this sum would be divided by the number of students who took the examination. A batting average would be computed by adding all the hits and dividing by the total number of times the individual was up to bat.

Returning to our example, we could compute the mean score by adding up the score each person chose (from 1 to 5 in our case) and divide by 10, the number of respondents. Therefore, our mean score is 2.3, as follows: $[(1 + 1 + 1 + 1 + 2 + 2 + 3 + 3 + 4 + 5) / 10 = 2.3]$ Before computing the mean score, we knew, based only on our observation of the frequency table, that many people didn't feel very susceptible to skin cancer. By computing the mean score, we can be much more precise and state that, on average, respondents tend to disagree they are susceptible to skin cancer. The mean score is important for two reasons. First, it is the most sensitive of all measures of central tendency that we consider. This means that a change in any single score affects the overall mean score of the group. The mean score is also important because this measure of central tendency is most frequently used in other computations of quantitative data analysis.

The *median* is a measure of central tendency specifying the exact middle score in a distribution. That is, half of the scores in the distribution lie above the median and half of the scores lie below it. Looking back at our example, we see that the number 2, associated with the response "Disagree" represents the median of our distribution. As you can see, four scores fall below this response category and four scores fall above it. As mentioned before, the median is not as sensitive as the mean score. Note that the me-

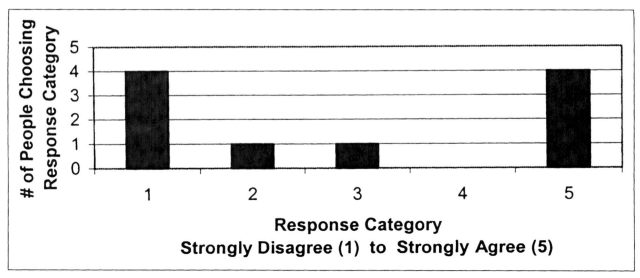

Figure 9.2 Bimodal Distribution

dian (2) does not change even if the two individuals who responded "Neutral" and the individual who responded "Agree" all had responded "Strongly agree." There would still be four scores above and four scores below the response category "Disagree." The mean score, on the other hand, would change from 2.3 to 2.8, a fairly significant jump.

The third and final measure of central tendency, the *mode*, simply represents the response given by the greatest number of individuals. In our example, the mode is "1." That is, more respondents (four in all) chose "Strongly Disagree" than any other answer. The mode is easy to compute, but the least sensitive of the measures of central tendency. Note that responses could vary in any number of ways, but as long as most people still responded "Strongly Disagree," the mode does not change. Although less sensitive than the other measures, the mode can still provide useful information. On occasion, you may find that your distribution has two modes, that is, a similarly high number of respondents providing answers in two response categories. We refer to such distributions as being *bimodal*. For example, if four people in our sample had chosen "Strongly Agree (5)" and four had chosen "Strongly Disagree (1)," with the remaining people choosing "Disagree (2)" and "Neutral (3)," then we would have a bimodal distribution with about half of the population believing they were highly susceptible to skin cancer and about half believing they weren't (see Figure 9.2).

Measures of Dispersion

In addition to measures of central tendency, it may also be beneficial to consider measures of dispersion. Although the central tendency measures provide information about how scores tend to cluster together, the measures of dispersion provide information about the variance of scores, or how spread out the scores tend to be. The easiest measure of dispersion to compute is the *range*, which is computed by subtracting the lowest score obtained from the highest score obtained, and then adding (1). In both of our figures, scores range between a low of (1) and a high of (5). Thus, we compute the range as [(5-1) +1 = 5]. As a measure of dispersion, the range, like the median and

Table 9.2 Calculation of Variance

Scores	Deviation from the Mean (step 1)	Squared Mean Deviation (step 2)
5	5 - 2.3 = 2.7	$2.7^2 = 7.29$
4	4 - 2.3 = 1.7	$1.7^2 = 2.89$
3	3 - 2.3 = .7	$.7^2 = .49$
3	3 - 2.3 = .7	$.7^2 = .49$
2	2 - 2.3 = −.3	$-.3^2 = .09$
2	2 - 2.3 = −.3	$-.3^2 = .09$
1	1 - 2.3 = −1.3	$-1.3^2 = 1.69$
1	1 - 2.3 = −1.3	$-1.3^2 = 1.69$
1	1 - 2.3 = −1.3	$-1.3^2 = 1.69$
1	1 - 2.3 = −1.3	$-1.3^2 = 1.69$

23 (Total)

[23/10 = 2.3] (Mean)

(Total) 18.1 (step 3)

(Variance) 18.1/10 = 1.81 (step 4)

mode, is a rather insensitive measure, as its computation is based on just two scores, excluding all others.

A more useful measure of dispersion, which (like the mean) is sensitive to all scores, is the *variance*. The variance of a distribution is calculated by subtracting the mean score from the actual scores obtained (step 1), squaring each result (that is, multiplying it by itself, step 2), adding together all squared results (step 3), and finally dividing the sum by the total number of scores (step 4). The computation of the variance is illustrated in Table 9.2, using the same distribution considered in Table 9.1 and Figure 9.1. The variance in our example is 1.81, a figure that indicates the average amount of dispersion around the mean. The higher the obtained value, the greater is the variability of scores obtained.

One final useful measure of dispersion is the *standard deviation* of the distribution. The standard deviation is similar to the variance in that it is sensitive to all scores obtained. The standard deviation is very useful because it indicates the pattern of dispersion. A relatively small standard deviation, for example, tells us that the respondents are very similar. A relatively large standard deviation, on the other hand, indicates there are large differences among respondents. Once the variance has been computed, it is relatively easy to calculate the standard deviation, because it is simply the square root of the variance. In our example, the standard deviation is the square root of 1.81, or 1.34. One reason the standard deviation is often used instead of the variance is that the standard deviation is expressed in the original unit of measurement. Additionally, the standard deviation is frequently used to describe samples and often incorporated in other, more advanced quantitative statistical computations.

Plotting the distribution of scores and calculating measures of central tendency and dispersion are likely to be useful tools for the basic quantitative data analyses you may conduct in a formative evaluation (to determine perceptions toward health risk messages) and a process evaluation (to determine if your health risk messages have been implemented appropriately). Distributions and measures of central tendency and dis-

Table 9.3 Frequency Table for Individuals Exposed to the Health Risk Message

Response Category	Number of Respondents Choosing This Answer
Strongly disagree	0
Disagree	2
Neutral/undecided	3
Agree	2
Strongly agree	3
Total	10

persion, however, are not sufficient for analyzing data associated with an outcome evaluation. Here, you need some additional tools, such as the *t* test.

t Tests

When conducting an outcome evaluation, we are often interested in testing group differences, including differences within the same group of respondents, for example, in their scores after receiving health risk messages as compared with those obtained before they were exposed to the messages. Alternatively, we might want to test for differences between two separate groups, comparing one group that received the health risk messages to another that did not. And in some cases, depending on the design selected for the outcome evaluation, both types of comparisons may be desired (e.g., pretest/posttest control group design). These comparisons can be made by using the *t* test.

To illustrate the use of the *t* test, let's assume our initial 10 respondents were never exposed to health risk messages focusing on skin cancer. Recall their mean response was 2.3, which indicated a relatively low rate of perceived susceptibility on a scale of 1 to 5. Now, assume we give the same statement ("I am likely to develop skin cancer") to a different group of 10 individuals, all of whom have been exposed to our health risk messages concerning skin cancer. Their responses to this item are provided in Table 9.3.

The mean score for this group of respondents who received the health risk messages is 3.6. The difference in the mean scores, 2.3 (from Table 9.1) versus 3.6 (from Table 9.3), suggests that the health risk messages had an effect on our respondents, leading to stronger perceived susceptibility (assuming both groups started out at an initial level of 2.3). But is this difference large enough, statistically speaking, to suggest it results from our intervention, assuming that exposure to the intervention was the only event related to this health risk that one group experienced while the other did not? The *t* test enables us to determine whether the mean of 3.6 from the group receiving the healthy risk message is significantly higher (meaning beyond that expected by chance) than the control group with a mean of 2.3. Table 9.4 illustrates the computation of the variance for this second frequency distribution. This is necessary to compute the *t* test.

To use the *t* test in our analysis, we begin by specifying two hypotheses, the research hypothesis and the null hypothesis. The research hypothesis states that the mean scores between the two groups are different; the null hypothesis states the mean scores between the two groups are the same (that is, no significant difference between them). If, in fact, the mean scores turn out to be significantly different (at the .05 level), then

Table 9.4   Calculation of Variance for Individuals Exposed to the Health Risk Message

Scores	Deviation from the Mean	Squared Mean Deviation
5	5 - 3.6 = 1.4	$1.4^2 = 1.96$
5	5 - 3.6 = 1.4	$1.4^2 = 1.96$
5	5 - 3.6 = 1.4	$1.4^2 = 1.96$
4	4 - 3.6 = .4	$.4^2 = .16$
4	4 - 3.6 = .4	$.4^2 = .16$
3	3 - 3.6 = -.6	$-.6^2 = .36$
3	3 - 3.6 = -.6	$-.6^2 = .36$
3	3 - 3.6 = -.6	$-.6^2 = .36$
2	2 - 3.6 = -1.6	$-1.6^2 = 2.56$
2	2 - 3.6 = -1.6	$-1.6^2 = 2.56$
36 (Total)		(Total) 12.4
[36/10 = 3.6] (Mean)		(Variance) 12.4/10 = 1.24 (step 4)

we reject the null hypothesis (that suggested no difference) and fail to reject (or sometimes we say, accept) the research hypothesis. The significance level we use is .05, which is the level most commonly specified by researchers in the social sciences. By setting the significance level at .05, we suggest we are 95% confident the null hypothesis is false. To put it another way, the possibility of the difference occurring as a result of chance or error is less than 5%.

The magnitude of the t statistic tells us whether the means are significantly different from each other, and its calculation is shown in Table 9.5. As you can see in Table 9.5, the value of t is 3.8. In short, the value of t is the mean difference between the groups divided by the variation that exists among the scores. Therefore, we first calculate the t statistic and then check a table to see whether this value is significant.

Now that we have a value for t, called the obtained t, what is the next step in the analysis? Recall our null hypothesis said no differences existed in the mean scores, and the research hypothesis said the mean scores were different. To determine which hypothesis to accept (and which to reject), we refer to a table listing the t distribution. Table 9.6 is used to determine whether the obtained t is significant, which again means occurring beyond chance. The numbers in the left-hand column in Table 9.6 are degrees of freedom, which represent the number of scores that may vary in a distribution. If there are five scores that sum to 20, for example, then four of these scores can vary, but one cannot; the last one is "reserved" to bring the sum to 20. The degrees of freedom in our example is determined by subtracting 2 from the total number of individuals surveyed $(20 - 2 = 18)$. The reason 2 is subtracted is because all but one number can vary in each of the two groups (one in the experimental group and one in the control group).

The numbers in bold on the top of Table 9.6 represent levels of probability. The numbers in the upper row are associated with a one-tail test and the numbers in the bottom row are associated with a two-tail test. You use a one-tail test if you specify the direction of change you expect, that is, you expect either a positive or negative change in attitudes. You use a two-tail test if you simply want to see if there is a change, but aren't

Table 9.5

Formula to compute t:

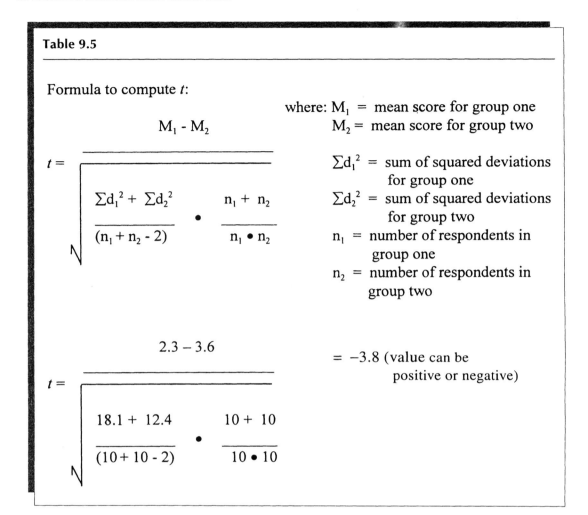

$$t = \cfrac{M_1 - M_2}{\sqrt{\cfrac{\sum d_1^2 + \sum d_2^2}{(n_1 + n_2 - 2)} \bullet \cfrac{n_1 + n_2}{n_1 \bullet n_2}}}$$

where: M_1 = mean score for group one
M_2 = mean score for group two

$\sum d_1^2$ = sum of squared deviations for group one
$\sum d_2^2$ = sum of squared deviations for group two
n_1 = number of respondents in group one
n_2 = number of respondents in group two

$$t = \cfrac{2.3 - 3.6}{\sqrt{\cfrac{18.1 + 12.4}{(10 + 10 - 2)} \bullet \cfrac{10 + 10}{10 \bullet 10}}}$$

= −3.8 (value can be positive or negative)

sure of its direction, positive or negative. Because we did not specify how or in which direction the scores would change, we use the bottom row of numbers, that is, the numbers for a two-tail test. Now we find the number that corresponds to 18 degrees of freedom (moving down the left hand column) and a probability level of .05 (moving across) and see that it is 2.101. Because the calculated value of t is −3.8, which exceeds ±2.101 (plus or minus 2.101), the difference in mean scores groups is deemed significant. Note that it doesn't really matter (for our purposes) if t is positive or negative, what matters is that it exceeds ±2.101. Therefore, we reject the null hypothesis that there are no differences between the groups and accept[1] (or fail to reject) the research hypothesis that the mean scores are different.

Another way of expressing this is to say that, given the value of the obtained t score, (3.8), we are 95% confident that the mean score differences are "real," and not the result of chance or error. To put it yet another way, there is less than a 5% chance the t score we obtained is the result of chance or error. If the calculated t score had been less than 2.101, we would have concluded that the mean score differences between groups might have been the result of chance or error. In this case, we would have accepted the null hypothesis, and concluded that, for our purposes, the means did not differ, at least statistically speaking.

Table 9.6 *t Distribution*

	Level of Significance for One-Tailed Test					
	.05	.025	.01	.005	.001	.0005
	Level of Significance for Two-Tailed Test					
df	.10	.05	.02	.01	.002	.001
1	6.314	12.706	31.820	63.657	318.309	636.619
2	2.920	4.303	6.965	9.925	22.327	31.599
3	2.353	3.182	4.541	5.841	10.215	12.924
4	2.132	2.776	3.747	4.604	7.173	8.610
5	2.015	2.571	3.365	4.032	5.893	6.869
6	1.943	2.447	3.143	3.707	5.208	5.959
7	1.895	2.365	2.998	3.499	4.785	5.408
8	1.860	2.306	2.896	3.355	4.501	5.041
9	1.833	2.262	2.821	3.250	4.297	4.781
10	1.812	2.228	2.764	3.169	4.144	4.587
11	1.796	2.201	2.718	3.106	4.025	4.437
12	1.782	2.179	2.681	3.055	3.930	4.318
13	1.771	2.160	2.650	3.012	3.852	4.221
14	1.761	2.145	2.624	2.977	3.787	4.140
15	1.753	2.131	2.602	2.947	3.733	4.073
16	1.746	2.120	2.583	2.921	3.686	4.015
17	1.740	2.110	2.567	2.898	3.646	3.965
18	1.734	2.101	2.552	2.878	3.610	3.922
19	1.729	2.093	2.539	2.861	3.579	3.883
20	1.725	2.086	2.528	2.845	3.552	3.850
21	1.721	2.080	2.518	2.831	3.527	3.819
22	1.717	2.074	2.508	2.819	3.505	3.792
23	1.714	2.069	2.500	2.807	3.485	3.768
24	1.711	2.064	2.492	2.797	3.467	3.745
25	1.708	2.060	2.485	2.787	3.450	3.725
26	1.706	2.056	2.479	2.779	3.435	3.707
27	1.703	2.052	2.473	2.771	3.421	3.690
28	1.701	2.048	2.467	2.763	3.408	3.674
29	1.699	2.045	3.462	2.756	3.396	3.659
30	1.697	2.042	2.457	2.750	3.385	3.646
50	1.676	2.009	2.403	2.678	3.261	3.496
100	1.660	1.984	2.364	2.626	3.174	3.390
∞	1.645	1.960	2.326	2.576	3.090	3.291

SOURCE: From Mary B. Harris, *Basic Statistics for Behavioral Science Research* (2nd ed.), p.157. Copyright © 1998 by Allyn & Bacon. Reprinted by permission.

Let's take this analysis one step further by reexamining our research and null hypotheses. Our research hypothesis states the mean scores would be different, but we do not specify how. That is, we do not specify which group's mean is higher than the other's. However, because our health risk messages are designed to increase respondent's levels of perceived susceptibility, we could have specified a direction, namely, that mean scores obtained after disseminating health risk messages would be higher than the mean scores prior to that time. In other words, our research hypothesis could have stated that the mean scores obtained from the group of individuals receiving the health risk messages would be higher than the mean scores obtained from the group of individuals not receiving the messages. Although the null hypothesis remains the same—that there is no difference between group means—the research hypothesis changes. Rather than merely suggesting the mean scores are different, the research hypothesis now suggests that the mean score obtained from the second group (the group of individuals receiving the health risk messages) is higher than the mean score obtained from the group of individuals not receiving the messages, suggesting higher levels of perceived susceptibility.

If this is our research hypothesis, we then use a one-tailed t test rather than a two-tailed t test. The computation of the t value is the same. To determine whether the one-tailed t- test result suggests the means are significantly different requires the use of the top row of numbers in Table 9.6 (recall that we used the bottom row earlier). The number corresponding to 18 degrees of freedom (moving down the left hand column) and a probability level of .05 (moving across) is 1.734. Because the obtained value of t of 3.8 is higher than 1.734, we again reject the null hypothesis suggesting no difference between means and accept (or fail to reject) the research hypothesis that the mean score obtained from the group receiving the health risk messages is significantly higher than the mean score obtained from the group not exposed to the messages.

This relatively simple analysis is valuable because it is evidence of the significant influence of your intervention on the audience's perceptions or behaviors. This type of data analysis helps funding sources and other key stakeholders see the worth of your project. And, as shown in these examples, this analysis is relatively easy to do.

▪▪ CONCLUSION

This chapter introduces some basic concepts of data analysis. The type of analysis you conduct ultimately depends on the types of questions asked and the subsequent information obtained. We first briefly looked at qualitative data analysis and then, more thoroughly examined quantitative data analysis. We initially discussed quantitative data analysis by reviewing three measures of central tendency (mean, median, and mode), and three measures of dispersion (range, variance, and standard deviation). The former represent how scores tend to cluster, and the latter indicate how scores tend to be distributed. We then proceeded to discuss the t test, a statistical test used to determine whether two mean scores differ significantly from each other. This is an extremely important test as it can indicate whether a single group of individuals changed from one time period to another (e.g., after an intervention). The t test can also be used to determine whether two unique groups of individuals are different at some time point (e.g., after one group receives the health risk messages and the other does not).

Although it is beyond the scope of this text to provide more than a cursory review of some basic analytic techniques, we hope the information in this chapter gives you the necessary vocabulary and tools to conduct data analyses, understand analyses conducted by others, and perhaps learn more sophisticated techniques. Table 9.7 lists definitions of terms used in this chapter, which we hope is a useful reference for you in your data analysis efforts.

CHAPTER 9

Table 9.7   Definitions

Analytical Term	Definition
Measures of Central Tendency	Provide information about the clustering of responses within a distribution.
Mean	The most important measure of central tendency, the mean is the score obtained by summing all respondents' scores and then dividing by the number of respondents. The mean score is sensitive to all scores in a distribution.
Median	The median is the middle score of a distribution, with half of all respondents' scores lying above it and half lying below it. The median score is not sensitive to all scores in a distribution.
Mode	The mode represents the most frequent score chosen by respondents. The mode is not sensitive to all scores in a distribution.
Measures of Dispersion	Provide information concerning how spread out the responses are within a distribution.
Range	The range is computed by subtracting the high score of a distribution from the low score and adding one. The range is not sensitive to all scores in a distribution.
Variance	The variance of a distribution is calculated by subtracting the mean score of the distribution from the respondents' scores, squaring each result, summing all squared results, and dividing the sum by the total number of scores. The variance is sensitive to all scores in a distribution.
Standard Deviation	The most important measure of dispersion, the standard deviation is computed by calculating the square root of the variance. This measure of dispersion is sensitive to all scores and furthermore, returns the variance to the original metric used.
Null Hypothesis	Statement suggesting, for example, that no difference exists between the two mean scores. If the obtained t score does not exceed some critical point, we fail to reject the null hypothesis, suggesting no differences exist between mean scores. If the obtained t score exceeds some critical point, we reject the null hypothesis, suggesting differences do exist between mean scores.
Research Hypothesis	Statement suggesting, for example, there is a difference between the two mean scores. If the obtained t score does not exceed some critical point, we reject the research hypothesis, suggesting differences do not exist between mean scores. If the obtained t score exceeds some critical point, we fail to reject the research hypothesis, suggesting differences do exist between mean scores.
Significance Level	The significance level is associated with the degree of confidence we have in the result of a statistical test such as the t test. Most commonly set at .05 in the social sciences, the significance level suggests there is less than a 5% chance the result of the t test (or some other test) results from chance or error.
t test	The t test is a statistical test used to determine whether the difference between two mean scores exceeds some critical point. The formula for conducting the t test is

$$t = \frac{M_1 - M_2}{\sqrt{\dfrac{\Sigma d_1^2 + \Sigma d_2^2}{(n_1 + n_2 - 2)} \cdot \dfrac{n_1 + n_2}{n_1 \cdot n_2}}}$$

where: M_1 = mean score for group one
M_2 = mean score for group two
Σd_1^2 = sum of squared deviations for group one
Σd_2^2 = sum of squared deviations for group two
n_1 = number of respondents in group one
n_2 = number of respondents in group two

▪▪ NOTE

1. Research scientists note that one can never "prove" a hypothesis. Therefore, they state that one can never "accept" a hypothesis. Rather, one can "fail to reject" a hypothesis. Put another way, if it turns out the data are "consistent with the hypothesis," then the research hypothesis "fails to be rejected." To be precise, hypotheses can either be "rejected" or "fail to be rejected." Colloquially, when a hypothesis is accepted, it means that the data are "consistent with the hypothesis" and the hypothesis has "failed to be rejected."

10

Getting the Message Out

F inally, you're ready to disseminate your campaign to the public. To this point, you have probably devoted a great deal of thought to (a) who your target audience is, (b) which topics are most important to your target audience (e.g., perceived susceptibility, perceived severity, self-efficacy, response efficacy), (c) which messages are most effective, (d) the length of your campaign, (e) methods of data collection and analysis, and perhaps (f) specific methods and channels for disseminating your message. This chapter focuses on how to get your message out so it has the desired impact.

There are numerous ways to get the message out to the target audience. Often campaigns incorporate a variety of activities disseminated through both interpersonal and mediated channels. Knowledge of the target audience, past research, and formative evaluation can all help identify the most appropriate methods and channels for your campaign. Take the bicycle safety campaign we discussed in Chapter 5. We've expanded that campaign here with specific channel and activity information for meeting its short-term objectives (Figure 10.1). Figure 10.1 shows that messages are to be disseminated through electronic mail (e-mail), a "Bicycle Safety Day" on campus, stories and public service announcements (PSAs) in the Healthy University student newspaper, and brochures (including a discount coupon making bicycle safety helmets more easily affordable). These channels and activities were identified by assessing previous successful campaigns and preferences noted by students in the formative research. We also took budgetary constraints into consideration and coordinated with other units on campus to develop this plan. Just as it was helpful to draw arrows from short-term objectives to middle-term objectives, here too, it is helpful to draw arrows from each activity to one or more of the short-term objectives. If an activity doesn't logically lead to the achievement of a short-term objective, then we must reconsider the purpose of the activity.

Of course, the number of specific objectives connected to each activity depends on the content of the messages included in each activity. In our example, student e-mail systems are used only to disseminate knowledge of bicycle safety signals, so each time a student's email account is accessed, a safety signal appears on the screen. Therefore, an arrow can be drawn from this activity to the short-term objective of increasing knowl-

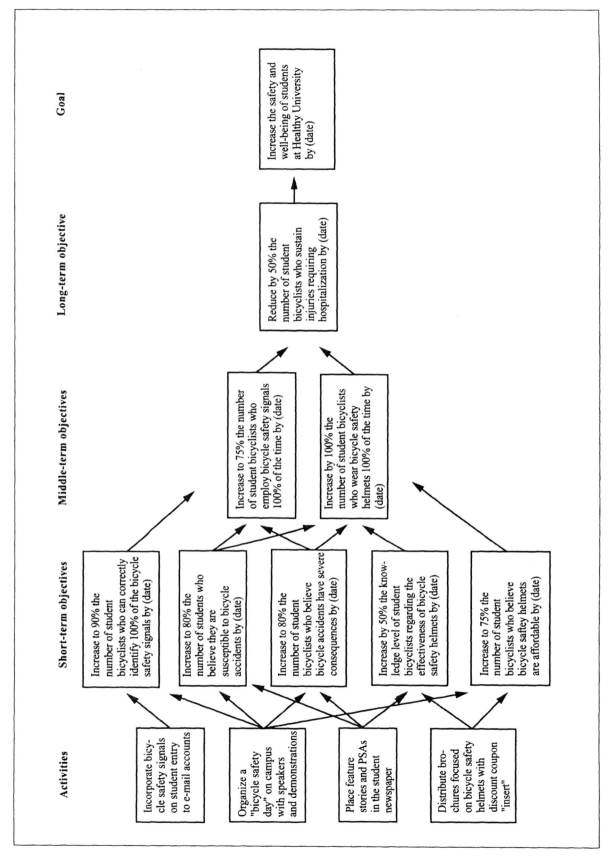

Figure 10.1 A Campaign Plan for Setting Goals, Objectives, and Activities

edge of bicycle safety signals, but not to any of the other objectives. Now consider the next activity, the campus-wide Bicycle Safety Day. An arrow appears leading from this activity to each of the short-term objectives, illustrating the assumption that each objective is addressed in some way by either the speakers or the planned demonstrations. The next activity focuses on placing feature stories and public service announcements in the student newspaper. Arrows are drawn from this activity to three short-term objectives addressing perceived susceptibility and severity as well as the efficacy of the recommended response, the bicycle safety helmet. The student newspaper, for example, may run a series of stories and PSAs focusing on the threat of bicycle injuries, highlighting students' susceptibility to accidents, and the severity of these accidents, while other stories might emphasize the effectiveness of safety helmets. Finally, brochures are to be distributed to Healthy University students at various locations around campus, such as the Healthy University Union, Student Health Clinic, dormitory lounges, libraries, and other areas where student traffic is heavy. Arrows are drawn from this activity to two short-term objectives, signifying the content of the brochure is directly related to the response and self-efficacy of bicycle safety helmets. Brochures, for example, may contain information about the design of bicycle safety helmets, show pictures of helmets damaged in accidents along with a testimonial from an individual who was saved from injury because of the helmet, and include the discount coupon enabling students to obtain a helmet at cost from the bicycle rental shop at the Union.

A PLAN OF ACTION ■■

Once activities have been specified, it is useful to form a detailed plan of action specifying when, where, why, how, and to whom you are disseminating messages. As an example, let's look at a different campaign, one focused on drinking among college students. Table 10.1 illustrates a plan of action for planning the dissemination of messages. Notice that the cost, contact name of coordinator of a particular phase of the campaign, and evaluation strategy are included in this plan.

The campaign is a relatively short, intense campaign, lasting only two months. Its main purpose is to decrease binge drinking (i.e., five or more alcoholic drinks in one sitting) and second, to reduce underage drinking among college students. Although the target of the campaign is college students, messages are directed toward the entire community, especially stores, bars, and restaurants that serve and/or sell alcohol to college students. Expanding the campaign into the community is necessary to ultimately change college students' behavior related to purchases of alcoholic beverages. This multimedia campaign utilizes a variety of channels, messages, and strategies to promote risk-reduction behaviors.

Table 10.1 shows that prior to the launch of the actual campaign is a one-month "community preparation" phase during which the community, students, and alcoholic beverage vendors are alerted to the upcoming campaign and encouraged to provide feedback to improve it (formative evaluation). Special efforts are made in this preparation phase to gain the cooperation of alcoholic beverage vendors. The plan indicates the activities by audience, the purpose of the activities, methods of evaluating their effectiveness, who is in charge of a particular phase, and the cost of the phase for budgetary purposes. Note that a variety of message strategies, media outlets, and evaluation methods are used. Also, note that during the month following the campaign, a summative or outcome evaluation phase will occur to assess effectiveness.

Table 10.1 Action Plan for "No More Excuses for Alcohol Misuses" Campaign

Month	Audience (who)	Activity (what)	Channel (how)	Location (where)	Purpose (why)	Evaluation	Coordinator	Cost
JAN	Community-at-large	Press releases, media interviews	Print, radio television, newspaper	Greater Lansing (MI)	Gain support for campaign; publicize launch of campaign	Telephone survey to assess awareness and attitudes	Lisa Jones 321-4567	$32 (postage, remainder volunteer)
	Students	Flyers on campus, Personalized e-mail	Print, electronic/internet	MSU Campus	Gain support for campaign, to promote school pride/good image	Electronic survey to assess awareness and attitudes	Pat Brown 345-9876	$300 (flyers)
	Alcohol vendors in area	Personalized letter	Print	Greater Lansing (MI)	Gain cooperation for minimizing binge and underage drinking	Enrollment as participant in campaign	Terry Smith 987-1234	$64 (postage)
FEB	Students, community, vendors	Public service announcements	Television (2) Radio (4) Newspaper (2)	Greater Lansing (MI)	Begin health risk message campaign to decrease misuse of alcohol	Telephone survey to assess awareness and attitudes	Steve Rice 567-8765	$2,000 (TV) $2,000 (radio) $300 (news)
	Students	Theatre troop	Live performances	Greeks MSU clubs	Begin health risk message campaign to decrease misuse of alcohol	Exit survey (paper/pencil) to assess attitudes & intentions	Skip Green 123-4321	No cost (volunteer)
	Alcohol vendors	Flyers and posters hung in establishments	Print	Greater Lansing (MI)	Begin health risk message campaign to decrease misuse of alcohol	Observation of venues that sell/serve alcohol—flyers/posters posted?	Erin Curtis 543-5678	$64 (postage)
MAR	Students, community, vendors	Public service announcements	Television (2) Radio (6) Newspaper (4)	Greater Lansing (MI)	Continue health risk message campaign to decrease alcohol misuse	Telephone survey to assess awareness and attitudes	Mark Johnson 345-3456	$2,000 (TV) $3,000 (radio) $600 (news)
	Students	Alcohol-free events	Peer educators, print (posters), live presentations	MSU Campus	Continue health risk message campaign to decrease alcohol misuse	Exit survey (paper/pencil) to assess attitudes, intentions, and behaviors	Susan Rivers 765-0987	$150 (mostly donations, volunteers)
	Community, students, vendors	Alcohol-free Day, (Information fair) (Theatre troop) (Skills workshops)	Live presentations, posters, media coverage, info booths, workshop	MSU Campus	Continue campaign to decrease misuse of alcohol Teach skills to resist pressure to binge drink	Exit survey (paper/pencil) to assess attitudes, intentions, and behaviors	Jill Roberts 432-9012	$2,000 (mostly donations, volunteers)
APR	Students	Outcome evaluation	Internet Telephone	MSU Campus	Evaluate effect of campaign on alcohol-related behaviors	E-mail survey, phone survey (attitudes/behaviors)	Bear Atkin 567-3210	$1,800 (final evaluation)

For a short, intense campaign such as this one, you may decide to break the activities down into weeks instead of months. The more precise and specific the plan of action is, the better. However, it is very important to remember this is just a plan. Be flexible! If one of the interim evaluations indicates a slogan or message isn't working, adjust it. If you get the opportunity to add some hip events, do so. Use this chart much as you would use a road map; allow yourself to enjoy the scenery and take some side trips if they look good.

■■ MESSAGE DISSEMINATION ISSUES

The remainder of this chapter focuses on the delivery of health risk messages and channel selection for those messages. As you read through these sections, remember there is no single correct way to disseminate your message. In the end, the decisions you make necessarily entail weighing the benefits and drawbacks of the various channels and selecting those fitting your campaign best.

There are several different channels you might select to disseminate your health risk messages, some interpersonal and others mediated. A health risk message disseminated from a counselor to a client at an HIV testing site is an example of an interpersonally based channel. The use of radio, television, newspapers, billboards, videos, and the Internet all typify mediated channels, because the messages go through some type of mass medium. Several factors should be considered when determining which channels to use in your campaign. They include (a) target audience preferences, (b) the purpose of the message, (c) message complexity, (d) the message source, (e) message accessibility, and (f) the availability of resources.

Target Audience Preferences

For effective dissemination, find out what channels your target audience wants to get its messages from. Do they want live presentations? Radio or television dramas? Brochures or pamphlets? Simply ask them as part of your formative evaluation. To be sure, target audience members do not pay attention to messages disseminated in a format or through a particular channel they are not receptive to. Rather, the format and channel should be selected based on their compatibility with the needs, past experiences, and values of the target audience (Rogers, 1995). The use of a print medium, for example, would be a poor selection for a target audience with an overall low literacy rate, or for a target audience comprised of young children. In these cases, it makes more sense to use an audiovisual or live (in-person) format. On the other hand, a printed message may be ideal for reaching a busy professional used to processing information in this format. Billboards may be the best way to urge motorists to slow down in construction zones. Be sure to obtain specific information in your formative evaluation, such as your audience's favorite radio stations, where they shop for groceries, or what clinics they attend, among other data.

Message Purpose

Your purpose should be carefully examined as you make decisions about how best to disseminate health risk messages to your target audience. Go back to the stages of change to figure out the specific purpose of your campaign. Is it to move people from precontemplation to contemplation? Contemplation to preparation? Preparation to action? Action to maintenance? Or, to address relapse issues? In some cases, for example, your purpose may be to create awareness of a particular issue, or in other words, to make the issue more salient to target audience members. This is a common strategy if the target audience is unaware of a particular threat; as a result, your objective is to move them from the precontemplation stage to the contemplation stage (Prochaska, DiClemente, & Norcross, 1992). Mediated forms of communication serve this purpose well and should probably be selected over interpersonal channels. In part, this is because mediated channels can repeat the message thereby increasing awareness, in a more cost-effective manner. The same reasoning applies if the purpose of your message is simply to disseminate facts or knowledge to target audience members.

Often, however, the objective is not simply to inform, but rather to persuade target audience members to engage in a particular behavior (e.g., wearing seat belts, applying sunscreen, exercising regularly), or refrain from particular behaviors (e.g., risky sexual practices, binge drinking, eating foods with a high fat content). In such cases, studies have demonstrated the effectiveness of using interpersonal communication channels along with mediated communication channels to move target audience members to behavior change (Rogers, 1995).

Message Complexity

The complexity of a message depends on your audience's stage of change. If you're simply trying to increase awareness, then a simple message probably works best. For simple messages, short PSAs or billboards are suitable. However, if you're moving people from preparation to action, detailed messages may be needed. In these cases, detailed videos, brochures, or pamphlets work better. Interpersonal, rather than mediated channels, may be used to disseminate particularly complex messages. Interpersonal channels enable the health educator to utilize multiple senses, obtain immediate feedback (if the receiver looks confused, the message can be repeated or restated), and engage in dialogue with the receiver as well as answer any questions that may arise.

Message Source

Although some messages are disseminated without explicit attachment to a source, it is much more common to see messages linked directly to specific sources (e.g., the Surgeon General's warning on packages of cigarettes) or a sponsoring agency (e.g., state health department advocating child immunizations). Therefore, consideration should be given to the source behind the message. The source should have a high degree of credibility, which may be defined as having expertise, trustworthiness, and dynamism. Even more important, to be viewed as credible, a source must be perceived as expert on the topic, either through study or personal experience. Earvin "Magic" Johnson, for example, may be perceived as a credible source for HIV prevention, but may be viewed quite differently for a topic such as testicular cancer.

A source also must be perceived as trustworthy. That is, the audience must see the source as someone who tells the truth and who cares about the audience. Finally, a dynamic source, or one with energy and charisma, is also perceived to be highly credible to an audience. It is worth noting that perceptions of source credibility vary from audience member to member. Furthermore, an individual perceived to have a high degree of credibility on one topic is not necessarily perceived as highly credible on another. Similarly, an individual with a high degree of credibility among one target audience may not be perceived as highly credible with another. The best way to determine who your target audience views as credible is to ask them.

One way to increase perceptions of trustworthiness (and hence, credibility) is to select a source very similar to members of the target audience. Several models of behavior change advocate the use of homophilous, or similar, others to deliver messages and model behaviors (see, for example, Bandura, 1977; Rogers, 1995; Rogers & Bhomick, 1971). Such individuals are immediately trusted by target audience members because they are perceived to be "just like me" and thus, "know what it's like to walk a mile in my shoes." Often, individuals from the target audience are trained and then, disseminate messages themselves. Peer education is an example of matching the source with target audience members. The only difference is that the source has some specialized knowledge (expertise) that audience members do not. In some cases, the source is a former member of a particular group, but still perceived to be credible. Examples of such sources include former prostitutes who educate current prostitutes about HIV prevention (Dorfman, Derish, & Cohen, 1992). Individuals who were formerly illiterate, obese, or addicted to alcohol or other drugs might similarly be used as message sources for their respective topics.

An even more narrow use of target audience members focuses on the use of opinion leaders to disseminate messages. An opinion leader is an individual able to influence the attitudes of others within a social system on a fairly consistent basis (Rogers, 1995). This strategy has been successfully used in some campaigns (see, for example, Kelly et al., 1991) and is beneficial in that the opinion leader is not only a trusted member of the target audience, but also a highly influential member of the group.

Message Accessibility

By accessibility, we mean the extent to which target audience members either have access to the message or are likely to access the message. Imagine, for example, that your target audience is comprised of high school students and the campaign topic is nutrition. There are numerous ways you might try to reach this audience—some are likely to be more accessible than others. Attempts to reach this group with print messages at major supermarkets, with public service announcements in the food or health section of the mainstream newspaper, or via an AM radio talk show focused on "nutrition for life" are not at all likely to be successful because these message channels are not usually accessed by the target audience. On the other hand, accessible messages for high school youth are more likely to be found at the corner convenience store, in the local underground newspaper, or on their favorite radio station, which is probably an FM music station.

At times, we may want to focus our efforts on disseminating messages restrictively, in places where access is only possible for members of the target audience. Consider, for example, using women's fitting rooms in clothing stores to promote an initiative focused on reducing domestic violence against women. The placement of these messages in women's changing rooms makes it accessible only to women (primary target audience members), and furthermore, gives them the time and privacy needed to process the information and perhaps even write down a telephone number or address. Another example of restrictive accessibility, this time focused on men as the primary target audience, concerns the dissemination of messages focused on testicular cancer. Men's showers at health clubs might provide the ideal setting for print messages (laminated, of course). In this case, target audience members can review the information in a private setting and in some situations, may even try out the recommended response (a testicular self-exam).

Resource Availability

You'll need to consider the resources at your disposal, including money, personnel, materials, and services or other tangible resources that may be donated or voluntarily given to your campaign. The resources devoted to a campaign dictate, in part, the type and number of formats and channels used; in some cases, where or when the message(s) may be disseminated; and the length of time the messages can be disseminated. As an example, one of the authors was involved with a campaign to disseminate messages about gun safety through radio PSAs. This campaign differed from many, however, because sufficient resources were available to purchase airtime from radio stations and as a result, we had some influence over when the PSAs were played. We felt it was important to disseminate these messages during morning and afternoon drive times, that is, those times when most people are driving to or from work and thus, most likely to hear the message. Media sources regularly allocate a certain amount of airtime to PSAs; however, when this is done strictly as a public service (as their name implies), program coordinators have much less control over when the message is disseminated. If you've ever had trouble sleeping, you've probably been exposed to one or more public service announcements airing in the wee hours of the morning. Unless your message is directed toward a target audience of insomniacs or third shift workers, however, its effectiveness may be compromised. Given the fact that many health campaigns have limited funding, the onus often falls on the program director to creatively design an intervention on a shoestring budget.

▦ SPECIFIC CHANNELS

Now let's take a more detailed look at three specific means of disseminating health risk messages, including print, audiovisual, and live presentations. Each is commonly used to disseminate health risk messages and each has its unique advantages and disadvantages. Comparing these may help you determine which methods are best suited for your campaign.

We're Going to Print

Health risk messages have been disseminated through a variety of print formats including pamphlets, public service announcements in newspapers and magazines, books, posters, billboards, table-tents, and even *Val-Pak* coupons. Printed materials have several advantages relative to other forms of mediated communication. First, printed materials are relatively inexpensive to produce and distribute and may be done so in a relatively short period of time. One of the authors was involved in a project where health risk messages were disseminated through *Val-Pak* coupons to 70,000 households for just over $2,000—a small price to pay for the possibility of reaching an entire community. Some print media, such as brochures, provide a good opportunity to disseminate complex messages because target audience members can take the time to read it at their leisure. They can process the information at their own pace and reread sections if necessary. Another benefit of brochures is that they can be passed on to other interested individuals. Printed messages can continue to be distributed over a long period of time, assuming the information doesn't change. Often, health educators can obtain printed materials at no cost from other organizations for use in their campaigns.

Although one of the most widely used channels to communicate health risk messages, the print medium is limited in its ability to transmit emotional tone and quality, which may be especially important for messages focused on perceived threat. Because individuals process more of what they read and see, graphics should be an integral part of a printed health risk message. Some print formats are limited to rather simple messages. The messages on billboards, for example, must be succinct because viewers have a very brief amount of time to read them.

Videotapes and Visual Media

Audiovisual formats can be very effective when they are produced with scripts, graphics, and/or music pertinent, relevant, and carrying the proper emotive tones for the target audience. Several different audiovisual formats may be used to disseminate health risk messages, including videos, television programs, and televised public service announcements, as well as computer games and the Internet. An audiovisual format allows the developer of the health risk message to incorporate many elements of a "real-life" portrayal. In a video focused on gun safety one of the authors helped create, individuals whose lives were deeply and directly affected by gun injuries provided moving testimonials about their experiences (Roberto, Meyer, Atkin, and Johnson, 2000). Audiovisual formats are particularly advantageous because recommended responses can easily be demonstrated or modeled. In the aforementioned gun safety video, one individual demonstrates how easily a trigger lock can be placed over the trigger guard of a gun, thereby preventing access to the trigger. Some audiovisual formats such as videos are also advantageous because, as brochures, they can be repeatedly used over an extended period of time.

Audiovisual health risk messages, however, are relatively complicated and costly to produce. As such, professional production companies that are locally owned and operated are good sources of assistance. We suggest local production houses in part because they may have greater knowledge of the target audience. Furthermore, logistical costs associated with production are lower with a locally operated organization. If limited resources preclude your contracting a professional production house, look to experts at your local university (professors or graduate students) seeking opportunities to collaborate with local health educators. Although the initial cost of producing a video is often relatively high, the cost to copy and distribute the end product is relatively low. So, if you can find some way to produce the video, the overall costs of this format can be significantly reduced.

Saturday Night Live

The live format has many advantages over print and audiovisual formats, including adaptability of the content, the potential for vicarious learning, interactive capabilities, and the possibility of real-time modeling of health behaviors. The live format is especially suited for health risk messages based on the EPPM framework because the intensity of the threat or elimination of it can be adjusted to fit the audience efficacy profile.

The major limitations associated with the live format include the development of the event, the availability of competent presenters or actors, and coordination of the logistics associated with the presentation.

Two common methods associated with the live format include the standard health education pedagogy and the use of educational theater. Using the standard health education pedagogy, individuals, peers, and/or panels deliver messages through lectures, speeches, seminars, classrooms, rallies, and face-to-face sessions. The intent of health education delivered through standard pedagogical procedures is not to be entertaining and/or dramatic, although many times this is attempted. Nor is it intended to be story-like or indirect in its purpose. The intent of this method is to indicate the problem and the recommended response. Peer education programs on most college campuses train students to disseminate health risk messages. Few peer educators are trained to discern the level of threat or efficacy in the target audience, nor are many trained to model behaviors. As such, these programs may have limited effectiveness because of the nature of the presentation and because most people do not like to be told what to do, that is, lectured.

A more effective method of delivery may be one that adopts entertainment parameters. Delivery must be viewed as a process of making the environment conducive to message acceptance. Thinking and striving to make the whole communication experience intimate, hypnotic, and sensuous helps accomplish this. In the 1970s movie *All That Jazz*, the lead character, actor Roy Scheider, played an eccentric theater director. Before every show he'd stand in front of a mirror and exclaim, "It's show time!" His idea was that whenever you go in front of an audience, you must remember they are there to be entertained and your attitude and delivery are key. Three adjectives used to describe the impact of such communicative environments are hypnotic, intimate, and sensuous. Some might use these adjectives to describe their experience with a print format; more do so with audiovisual formats such as television; but usually such adjectives are associated with live presentations.

Health educators should give some consideration to using entertainment when delivering health risk messages. Some may feel entertainment is inappropriate when delivering messages focused on serious subjects such as cancer, AIDS, and alcohol-related deaths. However, the definition of entertainment suggests it may be appropriate. Entertainment is defined as "that which engages the attention agreeably, amuses or diverts, whether it is private, as by conversation, or in public, such as theater" (Webster, 1999). This is not to say all health messages should engage the target audience "agreeably," or that it should "amuse." The purpose for this suggestion is that, as we work to develop and deliver health risk messages, we consider how the message engages (entertains) our target audience. Live presentations, such as theater performances, seem to be one method ideally suited for this purpose.

Educational theater seems appropriate for delivering live health risk messages grounded in the EPPM framework. Educational theater is becoming a popular delivery format that uses dramatic presentations to explore behaviors, emotions, and convictions common to many target audiences faced with health-related decisions. It combines the concepts of education within the framework of entertainment to form what has been called "edu-tainment." One of the authors has used live theater to address serious health issues related to sexuality for more than five years. What makes this work well is that the target audience is intimately involved in the entire process. Presenters are recruited not as actors or experts, but as key members of the target audience, who have a good deal of knowledge as to what is pertinent and relevant to the majority of individuals in the target audience. It is the responsibility of the health educator to establish the goals and objectives of the campaign, as well as ensure that the messages are theoretically grounded. Developing the content of the messages, however, including identification and intensity of the threat and the manner in which appropriate behaviors (response and self-efficacy) are portrayed, should be left to the members of the theater group (perhaps with additional input from the target audience). The health professional, however, should still assume responsibility for the accuracy of the information, as well as the inclusion of any sociodemographic variations the message might need to better match the target audience.

Live theater is advantageous when part of the message focuses on individuals' self-efficacy levels associated with a particular recommended response. Bandura (1977) suggests efficacy is related to performance accomplishments, physiological states, verbal persuasion, and vicarious experience. Each is inherent to, or can be added to, a live presentation. Participant modeling or performance desensitization, verbal persuasion, vicarious experience from viewing live models, and the physiological or emotional arousal that comes from relaxation, symbolic desensitization, and/or exposure, are all possible outcomes for a target audience viewing live theater. Even with an audience whose efficacy level is unclear, live theater can blend threat and efficacy delicately to minimize the chance of moving audience members into fear control rather than danger control processes.

SUMMARY ▪▪

Disseminating your health risk messages to target audience members is an extremely important aspect of the health campaign. Even the best messages are not likely to be effective if inappropriate channels are selected for dissemination. In this chapter, we stressed the importance of careful thought as a prelude to channel or format selection. To begin, an activity should be considered viable if, and only if, it logically leads to meeting one of the campaign objectives specified in the developmental plan. Many different activities may help meet your objectives. Those you ultimately select should evolve after considering the preferences of the target audience, the purpose, complexity, and source of the message, message accessibility, and last, but certainly not least, the amount of resources you can direct toward the campaign. Once you have selected the activities for your campaign, you may find it useful to develop a detailed plan that specifies the activity, along with the intended audience, the channel and format, the location, purpose, evaluation, activity coordinator, and cost. This plan serves as a road map to help you coordinate and manage the numerous challenges of directing a health communication campaign.

CONCLUSION ▪▪

You are now equipped to develop, plan, conduct, and evaluate a full-scale health risk communication campaign. Your campaign is theoretically based and grounded in your audience's needs and values. If you follow the steps outlined in this book and practice with the worksheets, you can develop health risk messages that work. You can also evaluate the effectiveness of your campaign. Congratulations! You now are equipped with the tools to be an Effective Health Risk Communicator.

CHAPTER 10

Appendix

A Brief Analysis of Empirical Fear Appeal Studies

OVERVIEW ⏹

This Appendix is for those interested in the academic research on fear appeals. Over the past 45 years, a large number of studies have examined how diverse variables influence reactions to fear appeals. In an effort to organize these widely disparate studies, we have adopted the traditional model of communication, source-message-channel-receiver, as an organizing framework.

SOURCE FACTORS ⏹

Source Credibility

In general, the degree of source credibility in a fear appeal significantly and positively influences retention of information (Williams, Ward, & Gray, 1985) and message acceptance (McCroskey & Wright, 1971; Powell & Miller, 1967). Occasionally however, credibility of the message is unrelated to message acceptance (Leventhal & Niles, 1964). No differences between expert and nonexpert sources emerged on fear appeal effectiveness in Stainback and Rogers (1983). Some studies found that credibility and strength of fear appeal interacted to influence outcomes. For example, Hewgill and Miller (1965) found the greatest attitude change occurred in the high credibility and high fear condition, but fear was most important. Furthermore, Powell and Miller (1967) found messages threatening individuals with social disapproval worked only when delivered by a highly credible source who was seen as trustworthy. With source credibility as a dependent variable, Smith (1977) found that stronger threat messages were associated with greater derogation of a source's credibility. In Leventhal and Niles (1964), those at risk for a health threat (smokers for whom the fear appeal is relevant) tended to discount the credibility of a fear appeal when compared to those not at risk (nonsmokers) (Leventhal & Niles, 1964). Overall, source credibility appears to be an important variable to consider when designing fear appeals.

Similarity

The findings for source similarity to target audiences in a fear appeal are mixed. Dabbs (1964) found that individuals were more persuaded by those more similar in coping style/esteem level to themselves. Likewise, Dembroski, Lasater, and Ramirez (1978) discovered that 6th to 8th graders were more persuaded by sources of a similar race to themselves. However, race did not have a main effect or interact with level of a fear appeal to influence persuasion for Rhodes and Wolitski (1990). Ramirez and Lasater (1977) found that Anglos were more persuasive than Chicanos regardless of fear level for 5th to 8th graders. Overall, the findings appear mixed for the effectiveness of source similarity—especially for race.

Relevance to Topic

No clear patterns have emerged for the influence of source relevance to topic in fear appeals. Fritzen and Mazer (1975) discovered the greatest amount of behavior change occurred when an alcoholic communicator gave a low fear message. However, they also found that retention of information was better for a high fear appeal delivered by a nonalcoholic communicator. However, none of these results was statistically significant.

▪▪ MESSAGE FACTORS

Argument Quality

Argument quality appears to be an important variable to consider when developing fear appeals. Rodriguez (1995), Gleicher and Petty (1992), and Smith (1977) all found that argument quality influenced processing of a fear appeal such that the stronger the argument, the greater the persuasiveness of a fear appeal.

Message Sidedness

There appears to be no clear differences between one- and two-sided messages in terms of fear appeal effectiveness (Ley, Bradshaw, Kincey, Couper-Smartt, & Wilson, 1974; Skilbeck, Tulips & Ley, 1977; Smith, Kopfman, Morrison, & Ford, 1993). Furthermore, fear appeal and message sidedness do not appear to interact to influence outcomes (only fear appeals were effective) (Stainback & Rogers, 1983).

Subliminal versus Supraliminal Messages

Stephenson (1993) manipulated fear appeals supraliminally and subliminally and discovered that the subliminal fear appeal produced the most message acceptance and the least maladaptive outcomes.

Vividness

Vividness of a message may be defined as "the extent that it is (a) emotionally interesting, (b) concrete and imagery-provoking, and (c) proximate in a sensory, temporal, or spatial way" (Nisbett & Ross, 1980, p. 45). In an overall review not limited to fear appeals, Frey and Eagly (1993) found vivid messages to be "less memorable and less persuasive than pallid messages" (p. 32). However, Sherer and Rogers (1984) discovered that fear appeals with greater emotional interest, concreteness, and proximity lead to stronger intentions to perform a recommended response (Sherer & Rogers, 1984). Rook (1986) discovered that when a health threat was immediate, there was no effect resulting from vividness (defined as case history/personal story vs. abstract/generalized to all women). However, when a health threat was distal, then the vividness of a message was effective in changing beliefs. No impact on health behaviors because of vividness was found, however (Rook, 1986). Similarly, Lemieux, Hale, and Mongeau (1994) found no differences resulting from their vividness manipulation, which was a comparison of a fear appeal with color photographs to one with black and white photographs.

Message Framing

Framing health-related information in a fear appeal as a loss if the recommended response is not followed, as opposed to a gain if the recommended response is followed, appears to yield a more persuasive message (Meyerowitz & Chaiken, 1987; Perkins & Scott, 1986; Robberson & Rogers, 1988). Similarly, negative messages were remembered better than positive messages for Reeves, Newhagen, Maibach, Basil, and Kurz (1991). However, Lemieux, Hale, and Mongeau (1994) found no differences in persuasiveness between loss versus gain frames. Similarly, McCroskey and Wright (1971) found no differences between punishment or reward messages.

In terms of other message framing issues, Powell and Miller (1967) discovered that social disapproval messages produced more attitude change than social approval messages (but only by a credible source). Smart and Fejer's (1974) results suggested that preventive messages produce more effect than change messages. Robberson and Rogers (1988) found that positive appeals to self-esteem (e.g., increased self-confidence) worked better than negative ones (e.g., feeling worthless). Finally, Shelton and Rogers (1981) determined that high empathy/high fear appeals worked the best for pro-environment actions.

Severity of a Threat Depictions

The severity of a threat can be described in terms of outcomes like symptoms, duration (length of suffering), how a threat impacts one's appearance, and how the threat interferes with one's activities (Prohaska, Keller, Leventhal, & Leventhal, 1987). Studies have shown that threats described as highly visible and disfiguring lead to stronger intentions to protect oneself (Klohn & Rogers, 1991). Bang (1993) found that negative physical consequences were more emotionally arousing and persuasive than legal consequences for an antidrunk driving fear appeal. The degree of pain described for a threat does not appear to affect intentions or behaviors (Dabbs & Leventhal, 1966).

Imminent versus Remote/Distal Threat

Fear appeals containing imminent and immediate threats appear to be more effective than ones emphasizing remote and distant threats (Chu, 1966; Klohn & Rogers, 1991). Additionally, threats viewed as more likely to happen now than in the distant future were seen as more serious (Kok, 1983). Neither the rate of onset for a health threat (gradual vs. sudden) nor suggestions about when to undertake a recommended behavior appear to have an impact on message effectiveness (Leventhal, Jones, and Trembly, 1966).

Target of the Threat

Powell (1965) discovered that messages threatening the family produced the most attitude change, closely followed by messages threatening the listener (messages threatening the nation were the weakest). Witte, Murray, Hubbell, Liu, Sampson, and Morrison (in press) found that members of collectivist cultures (Hispanics) were more frightened by fear appeals threatening the family and members of individualist cultures (African-Americans) were more frightened by messages threatening oneself than the reverse for each.

■■ INFORMATION ABOUT THE RECOMMENDED RESPONSE

Many, many studies have shown that information about the effectiveness of the recommended response and about one's ability to perform the recommended response leads to greater message acceptance under high threat conditions and rejection of fear appeals under low threat conditions (e.g., Rippetoe & Rogers, 1987; Rogers & Mewborn, 1976; Tanner, Day, & Crask, 1989; Witte, 1992b). Response efficacy and self-efficacy are such important message components, they have been incorporated into two fear appeal theories (PMT, EPPM). Some qualitative work is beginning to emerge that examines the degree of threat and efficacy depicted in public health campaigns. Kline (1995) found that breast self-examination pamphlets published by national organizations (National Cancer Institute, American Cancer Society) emphasized severity and susceptibility, but did not have adequate levels of response efficacy or self-efficacy. Similarly, in a study conducted along the Trans-Africa Highway in Kenya, Witte, Nzyuko, and Cameron (1995) discovered that HIV/AIDS prevention materials contained adequate levels of severity and susceptibility, but were weak on response and especially self-efficacy messages. The types of fear appeals found by Kline

(1995) and Witte, Nzyuko, and Cameron (1995) would be most likely to produce fear control responses resulting in the failure of a fear appeal to influence behaviors.

Order of Recommendations

The optimal position for message recommendations appears to be immediately after the fear-arousing message. Skilbeck, Tulips, and Ley (1977) found that fear-arousing messages immediately followed by recommendations were much more persuasive than recommendations given first or recommendations given much later. Similarly, the highest level of acceptance (though nonsignificant) toward a message emerged in Leventhal and Singer (1966), when the recommendations were given after the fear appeal, as compared to before or during the fear appeal. Finally, Harris and Jellison's (1971) study suggested that fear arousal followed by recommendations produced more persuasiveness than fear arousal alone.

Duration of Exposure to a Fear Appeal

Leventhal and Niles (1965) showed the longer the exposure, the more positive were the attitudes toward the message's recommendations and the greater were the perceived seriousness of a threat. Fear arousal was not affected by duration of exposure.

Repetition

The findings for repetitions of a message are mixed. Horowitz (1969) found that number of exposures (1 vs. 5) to a fear appeal had no effect on attitude changes. Kirscht and Haefner (1973) discovered that number of repetitions (1, 2, or 3) had no effect on intentions but did have an effect on behavior with more repetitions resulting in more behavior changes. Skilbeck, Tulips, and Ley (1977) determined that a single exposure to a fear appeal resulted in more persuasiveness than did multiple exposures (daily reminders).

CHANNEL FACTORS ■

Frandsen (1963) compared high and low fear appeals presented live, by television, and by audiotape. He found that media type did not significantly influence message acceptance. However, his results indicated that the high threat/live presentation was the most persuasive and the low threat/audiotaped fear appeal was the least persuasive. Janis and Mann (1965) found that those who role-played a fear-arousing message (a lung cancer victim receiving bad news) changed their smoking habits more than those who listened to the role-play session on audiocassette.

In terms of channel features, Leventhal and Trembly (1968) found that the larger the screen and the louder the sound was, the lower were perceived invulnerability, coping, and concentration, and the greater were the strength of emotions (disgust, impotence, egotism, depression, avoidance). There was no effect on intentions resulting from screen size or sound volume.

■■ RECEIVER FACTORS

Gender

There appears to be no effect due to gender on acceptance of fear appeal recommendations (Insko, Arkoff & Insko, 1965; Leventhal, Jones, & Trembly, 1966; Rhodes & Wolitski, 1990). However, Struckman-Johnson, Gilliland, Struckman-Johnson, and North's (1990) study suggested that males were more persuaded by condom ads than females.

Self-Esteem

Those people with high self-esteem appear to accept fear appeal recommendations and take protective action compared to those with low self-esteem (Leventhal & Trembly, 1968; Ramirez & Lasater, 1977). In addition, those individuals with low self-esteem appear to adopt more maladaptive coping strategies (e.g., fatalism, denial) than individuals with high self-esteem (Leventhal & Trembly, 1968; Rosen, Terry, & Leventhal, 1982). Dabbs and Leventhal (1966) found that those with high self-esteem complied only in the high fear condition (although compliance was low overall). Leventhal and Perloe (1962) found that high self-esteem individuals were more persuaded by a positive message while low self-esteem persons were more persuaded by a negative message.

Locus of Control

Beck and Lund (1981) found that those with an external health locus of control with high susceptibility perceptions reported flossing their teeth the most. Health locus of control did not interact with fear appeal level to influence behaviors. Burnett (1981) also found that those individuals with an external locus of control were more persuaded by any fear appeal message when compared with those with an internal locus of control (no interactions with strength of fear appeal).

Trait Anxiety

In a replication of Boster and Mongeau (1984), the effects of trait anxiety on fear appeal persuasiveness were assessed in Witte and Allen (in press). Eleven investigations measured either trait anxiety or similar concepts (e.g., repression-sensitization, coper/avoider).[1] The results indicated that low anxiety individuals are slightly more persuaded by fear appeals than high anxiety individuals ($r = -.049, p < .05, N = 1,641, X^2 = 15.07$). There appeared to be no interaction between level of fear appeal and trait anxiety. Recent research has shown that trait anxiety also appears to influence the degree of defensive avoidance produced by a fear appeal (Witte & Morrison, 2000).

Relevance of Study Topic to Receiver

Four studies have shown that greater resistances to fear appeals emerge for those most in need of self-protective behavior change (Berkowitz & Cottingham, 1960; Leventhal & Niles, 1964; Leventhal & Watts, 1966; Liberman & Chaiken, 1992). For example, Leventhal and Niles (1964) found that smokers exhibited greater resistances to an antismoking communication when compared with nonsmokers. Similarly, Leventhal and Watts (1966) found that light smokers who felt vulnerable to harm were most persuaded by fear appeals but heavy smokers who felt invulnerable to harm were least persuaded. Liberman and Chaiken (1992) also found greater fear and less message acceptance for those to whom the message was relevant when compared with those to whom the message was irrelevant. Additionally, they discovered biased message processing (discounting, more defensive reading, more critical) for high relevance persons, but no defensive inattention to the message. In contrast, Beck and Davis (1978) found that relevance of topic and interest level of subject did not influence persuasiveness; only fear level did.

Defensive Processing

One relatively new way to look at fear appeals is through the message processing models of Chaiken (systematic-heuristic model, 1980, 1987) and Petty and Cacioppo (elaboration likelihood model, 1986). Though there are differences between the models, each model suggests two general routes to persuasion. When persons are motivated and able to process a message, they centrally or systematically process the message by carefully evaluating the message's arguments and then make their decisions. Messages that are processed via a central or systematic route can be processed in either a biased or unbiased manner (e.g., accurate vs. inaccurate). In contrast, when persons are not motivated and/or are unable to process a message, they process it peripherally or heuristically and evaluate messages on the basis of cues (e.g., number of arguments in a message) or heuristics (i.e., mental models; e.g., my neighbor uses aspirin, so I will, too) when making decisions. Typically, researchers look at the degree of message-relevant thoughts to determine whether systematic/central processing or heuristic/peripheral processing occurred. Greater message-relevant thoughts indicate systematic/central processing and fewer message-relevant thoughts indicate heuristic/peripheral processing.

Thus far, the research testing these dual process models has had mixed results. Some scholars have found that strong fear appeals promote systematic/central processing (Liberman & Chaiken, 1992), although others have found that strong fear appeals promote heuristic/peripheral processing (Hale & Mongeau, 1995; Jepson & Chaiken, 1990). A possible explanation for these results is that strong fear appeals promote biased defensive systematic/central processing and not the "normal" kind of systematic/central processing tested for in the two studies finding support for heuristic/peripheral processing (i.e., Jepson & Chaiken, 1990). For example, Liberman and Chaiken (1992) found that fear appeals were processed in a defensively biased manner such that threatening information was critically evaluated but reassuring information was not (Liberman & Chaiken, 1992). For high relevance subjects (those at risk for harm by the health threat), the defensive systematic processing was even more pronounced. Other researchers also have found selective and biased processing of fear appeals (Alvaro & Burgoon, 1995).

It may be that this biased defensive systematic/central processing masquerades as heuristic/peripheral processing because of the types of message processing measures used in the two studies finding evidence for heuristic/peripheral processing. For example, Hale and Mongeau (1995) defined degree of message processing as the proportion of positive thoughts to total thoughts about the fear appeals. However, if individuals were engaging in defensive systematic/central processing, then a potentially more accurate measure of systematic processing (defined as message-relevant thoughts) might be the proportion of *negative* thoughts to total thoughts. If this type of measure had been used, then it appears that Hale and Mongeau's (1995) results would have flipped with the strong fear appeal promoting more defensive systematic/central processing than the low fear appeal, as indicated by the number of negative thoughts toward the fear appeal. In Jepson and Chaiken (1990), degree of message processing was determined by assessing the total number of message-related thoughts listed as well as the number of planted errors alluded to by the subject. This latter measure is likely to indicate the degree of *unbiased* message processing, in that it tests whether a subject detects errors, but it does not give the degree to which *biased* message processing occurs. Their results indicated that there was no relationship between the strength of the fear appeal and number of message-related thoughts. Interestingly, there was a significant negative relationship between strength of the fear appeal and detection of errors. This finding would indicate that strong fear appeals result in less unbiased message processing, but it does not indicate whether biased defensive systematic processing occurred. It is plausible that subjects detected errors only for threatening information, but not for reassuring information. This type of pattern would indicate biased systematic processing.

Finally, Gleicher and Petty (1992) found a marginal interaction ($p < .07$) between fear appeal (moderate vs. low), argument quality (strong vs. weak), and response efficacy (whether a crime prevention program was successful).[2] Specifically, they found that, regardless of response efficacy level under low fear conditions, strong arguments were more persuasive than weak arguments. Under moderate fear conditions, a similar pattern emerged for low efficacy individuals where strong arguments were more persuasive than weak. However, for high response efficacy people under moderate fear conditions, strong and weak arguments were both very persuasive. Gleicher and Petty (1992) concluded that because the high response efficacy/moderate fear group did not differentiate between strong and weak arguments, the message must have been peripherally processed. However, another plausible interpretation of these results is that the high response efficacy/moderate fear group engaged in defensive systematic/central processing where reassuring arguments (even if they were weak) were bolstered, and threatening arguments were criticized. Overall, it is unknown whether the lack of differentiation between strong and weak arguments was the result of peripheral processing of the fear appeal or biased systematic processing. Further research is needed on this point.

Volunteer and Choice Status

Overall, volunteers are more persuaded by fear appeals than nonvolunteers (Horowitz, 1969; Horowitz & Gumenik, 1970). Furthermore, as strength of the fear appeal increases, so does message acceptance by volunteers and nonvolunteers allowed choice (they were allowed to choose among multiple experiments) (Horowitz & Gumenik, 1970).

Miscellaneous Individual Differences

A variety of personality factors appear to influence whether a fear appeal is persuasive. Highly misanthropic people (cynically hostile, distrustful) (Alvaro & Burgoon, 1995), conservative white middleclass consumers (Burnett & Oliver, 1979), children of high social status (Haefner, 1965), students with high aptitude scores (Insko, Arkoff, & Insko, 1965), and depressed and antisocial people (Self & Rogers, 1990) are not persuaded by fear appeals. In contrast, fear appeals tend to be more effective for older liberals and older blue-collar blacks (Burnett & Oliver, 1979), children of low social status (Haefner, 1965), and students with low aptitude scores (Insko, Arkoff, & Insko, 1965).

An individual's need for cognition appears to interact with level of threat and recommendations to influence intentions (Stout & Sego, 1994). Similarly, uncertainty orientation (the degree of motivation one has to resolve uncertainty) appears to interact with threat and efficacy such that those with a high uncertainty orientation are more likely to seek health information as the level of threat and efficacy in a fear appeal increases (Brouwers & Sorrentino, 1993). Some studies showed that regardless of age, gender, ethnicity, or group membership, the stronger the fear appeal, the more persuasive it was (Kirscht, Becker, Haefner, & Maiman, 1978; Rhodes & Wolitski, 1990).

MISCELLANEOUS FEAR APPEAL FACTORS ▪

Irrelevant Situational Fear

Mixed findings have emerged for the type of fear aroused—be it relevant or irrelevant to the fear appeal. Fear arousal unrelated to the fear appeal increased persuasiveness for Lundy, Simonson, and Landers (1967). However, Gleicher and Petty (1992) found no differences between relevant versus irrelevant fear conditions for message processing, and Simonson and Lundy (1966) discovered that any type of fear led to more positive attitudes.

False Physiological Feedback

Any type of arousal, actual or false (subjects were told they were aroused), appears to improve persuasiveness—regardless of the affective label it is given (Beck, 1979; Giesen & Hendrick, 1974; Hendrick, Giesen, & Borden, 1975; Schwarz, Servay, & Kumpf, 1985).

Subjective Expected Utilities

Using a rational decision-making perspective, Sutton and colleagues have obtained mixed results in tests of a Subjective Expected Utility model. Sutton and Hallett (1988) found the (a) utility of experiencing a health threat (e.g., the degree to which one cares about being harmed) and (b) the probability difference (the difference between experiencing the health threat minus the decrease in the perceived probability of experiencing the health threat if the recommended response is adopted) led to stronger intentions to quit smoking, but that (c) confidence (whether one thinks s/he can succeed in performing the recommended response) and (d) fear arousal were unrelated to intentions. In a three-study report, Sutton and Hallett (1989a) obtained mixed findings where utility never influenced intentions, confidence always positively influenced intentions, and fear arousal and the probability difference positively influenced intentions in two out of three studies. Similarly, the probability difference and fear significantly and positive influenced intentions to wear seatbelts in Sutton and Hallett (1989b). In contrast, confidence and fear positively influenced intentions to quit smoking in Sutton and Eiser (1984). Overall, the model has not fared well. Sutton and Eiser (1984) concluded in one study that there appeared to be "no evidence for the multiplicative combination of utilities and subjective probabilities" suggested by the SEU (p. 14). Furthermore, it appears that fear offers the most reliable influence on intentions, even though it is unrelated to the SEU model.

Multiple Affective Responses

Several studies have found that fear appeals produce multiple affective responses beyond fear (Dillard, Plotnick, Godbold, Freimuth, & Edgar, in press; Kirscht & Haefner, 1973; Kohn, Goodstadt, Cook, Sheppard, & Chan, 1982; LaTour & Pitts, 1989; Leventhal & Trembly, 1968). For example, Dillard, Plotnick, Godbold, Freimuth, and Edgar (in press) found that although the strongest emotion produced by fear appeals was fear, fear appeals also produced significant levels of surprise, puzzlement, anger, and sadness. Other outcomes of fear appeals include irritation (Kirscht & Haefner, 1973), disgust and feelings of impotence (Leventhal & Trembly, 1968), tension and energy (LaTour & Pitts, 1989), and varying degrees of emotional upset including anxiety, loss of pleasure, and depression (Kohn, Goodstadt, Cook, Sheppard, & Chan, 1982).

∷ SUMMARY

Overall, under all cases, the stronger the fear appeal, the greater the fear and perception of risk and the more persuasive a fear appeal is (Boster & Mongeau, 1984; Witte & Allen, 1996). Furthermore, several studies suggest that recommendation messages alone are less effective than recommendations with fear appeals (Harris & Jellison, 1971). Thus, it appears the combination of high threat and high efficacy messages produce stable and strong levels of attitude, intention, and behavior change. Fear appeals without efficacy messages or efficacy messages without fear appeals appear to be less persuasive.

When conducting a fear appeal study, it is critical to carefully define and make constructs operational. Furthermore, it is important to not only assess attitudes, intentions, and behaviors (i.e., danger control responses) but fear control responses, too (such as defensive avoidance, denial, and reactance). Throughout this book you are given clear definitions and questionnaire items useful in research studies.

NOTES ■■

1. Given Witte and Morrison's (2000) finding that previous fear appeal reviews examining the influence of trait anxiety on outcomes had inadvertently switched the high and low ends of scales measuring related constructs, great care was made to ensure the directionality of scales and labeling of anchors was accurate in Witte and Allen (in press). For example, sensitizers, high anxiety individuals, and copers all score high on trait anxiety scales; repressors, low anxiety individuals, and avoiders all score low on trait anxiety scales. See Witte and Morrison (2000) for complete review of the literature.

2. This interaction should be viewed cautiously as the manipulation check failed for response efficacy, indicating no differences between high and low response efficacy messages.

Glossary

The following are definitions and examples of the important variables found in most health behavior change models in the health risk message literature. See chapters 2, 3, 4, and 5 for descriptions of how these variables work together theoretically.

Attitudes
An evaluation of an object, recommended response, or a belief. For example, "computers are good; too much information is bad; anything that takes time is undesirable, are all attitudes.

Barriers
Anything that inhibits one from carrying out a recommended response, such as cost, time constraints, language difficulties, cultural differences, and so on. Some researchers see barriers as the inverse of self-efficacy, because barriers inhibit one's perceived ability to carry out a recommended response. Therefore, one can think of barriers as "barriers to self-efficacy." Examples of barriers for the NN/LM might be a lack of computer skills, cost, embarrassment, language issues, cultural issues, and so on.

Behaviors
The actual action carried out. For example, did you or did you not use the Internet daily last week?

Benefits
The rewards or positive consequences occurring as a result of performing a recommended response. Do people see any benefit to performing a certain behavior? Benefits are somewhat similar to response efficacy.

Cues to Action, External and Internal
Examples of external cues include public service announcements and informational flyers. Some internal cues are symptoms of an illness, such as an itchy or bleeding mole. Cues are pieces of information that trigger decision-making actions.

Danger Control
A process individuals engage in when they believe they are at risk for a serious or significant threat (i.e., high perceived threat), they believe they are able to effectively avert it from occurring (i.e., high perceived efficacy) and are motivated to control the

danger or threat. When people are motivated to control the danger, they change their attitudes, intentions, and behaviors. These changes result in the individual's adoption of behavioral recommendations in the message and subsequent enactment of the behavioral recommendations.

Defensive Avoidance
A motivated resistance to a recommended response, usually occurring at the subconscious level. Characterized by a lack of attention or remembrance of a particular concept, threat, or recommended responses. For example, the following are typical defensive avoidant responses: "It's too overwhelming, I'm just going to not think about it"; "I don't want to know anything about X, I'm just going to block out anything I hear about it." Defensive avoidance occurs when one perceives a significant and relevant threat, but believes nothing he or she can do will effectively avert the threat.

Efficacy
The effectiveness, feasibility, and ease with which a recommended response impedes or averts a threat. For example, can your audience easily and effectively find the information needed to avert a threat? Efficacy is comprised of two dimensions, response efficacy and self-efficacy. See these definitions below.

Fear
A high level of emotional arousal caused by perceiving a significant and personally relevant threat. Fear motivates both protective and maladaptive action, depending on the circumstances. For example, sometimes fear motivates one to seek out information. However, sometimes fear causes people to deny they are at risk for experiencing a threat or to defensively avoid a threat and thereby ignore recommended responses. Fear can be one of the most powerful influences on behavior if it is channeled in the right direction.

Fear Control
When people believe they are at risk for a serious or significant threat (i.e., high perceived threat), but they believe they are unable to perform the recommended response or they believe the recommended response to be ineffective (i.e., low perceived efficacy), then they focus on controlling their fear about the threat. When people control their fear they do not control the actual danger. Instead, they control their fear by denying they are at risk for the threat, defensively avoiding the threat, or reacting angrily toward those trying to help them.

Intentions
Your plans to carry out a recommended response or do a certain thing. For example, "I intend to use the Internet daily." Intentions are often used as proxies for actual behavior.

Reactance
Another form of motivated resistance where one becomes angry at an issue or source and reacts against a recommended response. Typically characterized by perceptions of manipulation (e.g., "they're just trying to manipulate us into using this stuff; it doesn't really make a difference") or message/issue derogation (e.g., "this stuff is stupid; I know all I need to know"). Reactance occurs when one feels threatened but feels unable to do anything to effectively avert a threat (e.g., "I guess it's important to have up-to-date information, but there's no time and no money for me to get what I need.").

Response Efficacy
The degree to which the recommended response effectively averts the threat. Sometimes response efficacy is called "outcome expectations," and answers the question, if you perform a certain behavior, what do you expect the outcome to be?. For example, do people believe condoms prevent HIV transmission? Do people believe that having current medical information prevents harm to patients?

Self-Efficacy The degree to which the audience perceives they are able to perform the recommended response to avert the threat. Sometimes self-efficacy is called "efficacy expectations," and answers the question, what do you expect will happen if you attempt to perform a certain behavior? For example, do people believe they can use condoms to prevent HIV transmission? Do people believe they are really competent and able to access the information needed to make good medical decisions?

Severity The magnitude of harm expected from a threat. The significance or seriousness of a threat. The degree of physical, psychological, or economic harm that can occur. For example, is AIDS severe and serious? Is there a danger in not having up-to-date information?

Social Marketing The use of marketing principles and ideas to "sell" a pro-social idea or belief. This approach promotes the use of market research to discover important demographic and psychographic characteristics of one's target audience. Then it uses the Four Ps of marketing to sell the concept: product (the behavior or the product you want the target audience to adopt), price, promotion, and place (or positioning). This is a popular approach used in many outreach campaigns, but it is important to note that social marketing is an approach, and not a theory. Thus, it is best used in conjunction with a theory that offers guidance on the variables to study and how these variables work together to produce desired outcomes.

Stages of Change A classification scheme that suggests five stages to the performance of a behavior, namely, Precontemplation, Contemplation, Preparation, Action, and Maintenance. For example, people are in different stages of readiness with regard to given behaviors. Different persuasive strategies are needed in the different stages of change. It is important to determine your client's or audience's stage of change before developing a campaign. For example, if your audience is completely unaware of certain technological innovations, they have not begun to even consider using such innovations and are in the precontemplation stage. An awareness and knowledge campaign is most appropriate for this target group to move them from the precontemplation stage to the contemplation and preparation stages. A motivational campaign is used to move people from the contemplation and preparation stages to the action and maintenance stages.

Subjective Norm One's motivation to comply with what one believes his or her important referents believe. Notice this definition has two parts. First, your subjective norm is based on what you believe your significant others believe (note that the focus is on what you believe they believe, not what they actually believe). The more you are motivated to comply with a certain significant other or referent, the stronger the subjective norm. For example, if you are motivated to comply with your boss and your boss thinks it's a good idea that you utilize up-to-date information sources, then your subjective norm is strong for you to utilize up-to-date information sources.

Susceptibility The likelihood that a specific person or audience will experience a threat. The degree of vulnerability, personal relevance, or risk of experiencing a threat. For example, am I susceptible to AIDS? Are you at risk for falling behind in current medical knowledge?

Threat A danger or harmful event existing in the environment of which people may or may not be aware. For instance, a lack of pertinent information may be a threat, because this lack may cause harm to a patient. A threat is comprised of two dimensions: severity and susceptibility. See the definitions of these terms in this Glossary.

Worksheets

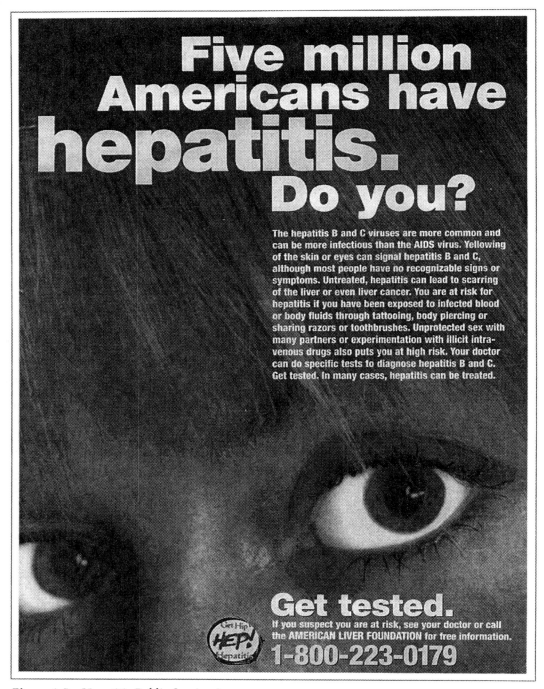

Figure 1.5 Hepatitis Public Service Announcement
SOURCE: Reproduced with permission, American Liver Foundation.

WORKSHEET 1: ANALYZING HEALTH RISK MESSAGES

Hepatitis—American
Liver Foundation

Name: _____

Date: _____

Course: _____

Section: _____

Due:_____

Professor: _____

Instructions: On the facing page is a health risk message. Please examine it carefully and answer the following questions completely. When asked to explain your answer, provide the reasons you answered the question the way you did.

1. What is the threat in this health risk message?

_____

_____

_____

2. Is the threat social, economic, spiritual, physical, or something else? Please explain.

_____

_____

_____

3. Is the threat implicit or explicit? Please explain.

_____

_____

_____

4. What is the recommended response?

_____

_____

_____

5. Is the recommended response implicit or explicit? Please explain.

_____

_____

_____

6. Are there any special colloquialisms in this health risk message that might not be understood by members of other cultures? Please list and explain.

_____

_____

_____

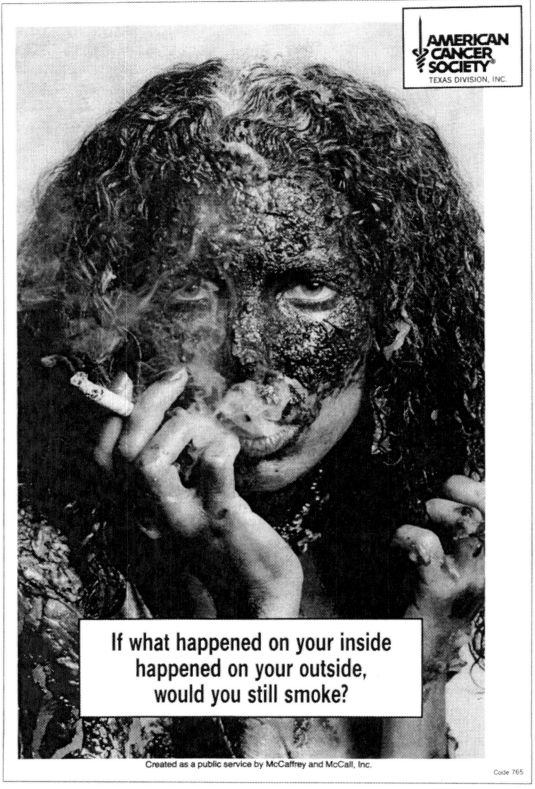

AMERICAN
CANCER
SOCIETY®
TEXAS DIVISION, INC.

If what happened on your inside
happened on your outside,
would you still smoke?

Created as a public service by McCaffrey and McCall, Inc.

Code 765

Figure 1.6 "If what happened on your inside happened on your outside"
SOURCE: Reprinted by the permission of the American Cancer Society, Inc.

WORKSHEET 2: ANALYZING HEALTH RISK MESSAGES

Smoking PSA
"If what happened on your inside
happened on your outside. . ."

Due: _____

Name: _____
Date: _____
Course: _____
Section: _____
Professor: _____

Instructions: On the facing page is a health risk message. Please examine it carefully and answer the following questions completely. When asked to explain your answer, give reasons describing why you answered the question the way you did.

1. What is the threat in this health risk message?

_____
_____
_____

2. Is the threat social, economic, spiritual, physical, etc.? Please explain.

_____
_____
_____

3. Is the threat implicit or explicit? Please explain.

_____
_____
_____

4. What is the recommended response?

_____
_____
_____

5. Is the recommended response implicit or explicit? Please explain.

_____
_____
_____

6. Are there any special colloquialisms in this health risk message that might not be understood by members of other cultures? Please list and explain.

_____
_____
_____

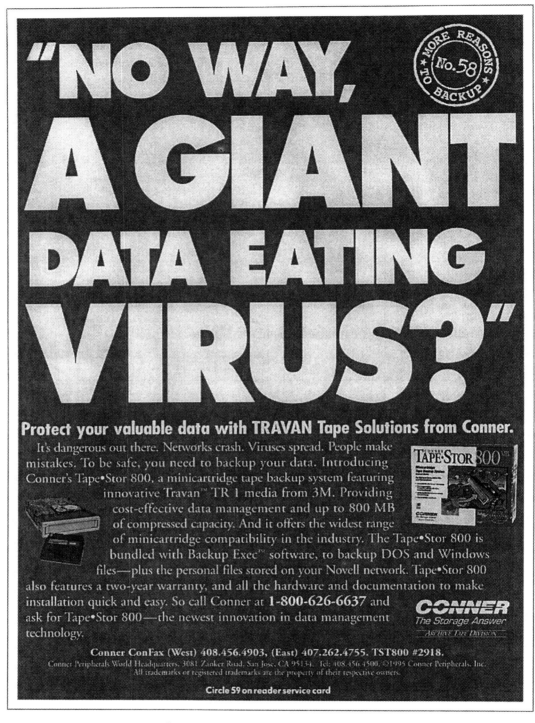

Figure 1.7 "No way, a giant data eating virus"
SOURCE: Reproduced with permission of Conner Peripherals, Inc.

WORKSHEET 3: ANALYZING HEALTH RISK MESSAGES

*"No Way, A Giant
Data Eating Virus!"*

Name: _____

Date: _____

Course: _____

Section: _____

Due: _____

Professor: _____

Instructions: On the facing page is a health risk message. Please examine it carefully and answer the following questions completely. When asked to explain your answer, provide the reasons you answered the question the way you did.

1. What is the threat in this health risk message?

_____

_____

_____

2. Is the threat social, economic, spiritual, physical, or something else? Please explain.

_____

_____

_____

3. Is the threat implicit or explicit? Please explain.

_____

_____

_____

4. What is the recommended response?

_____

_____

_____

5. Is the recommended response implicit or explicit? Please explain.

_____

_____

_____

6. Are there any special colloquialisms in this health risk message that might not be understood by members of other cultures? Please list and explain.

_____

_____

_____

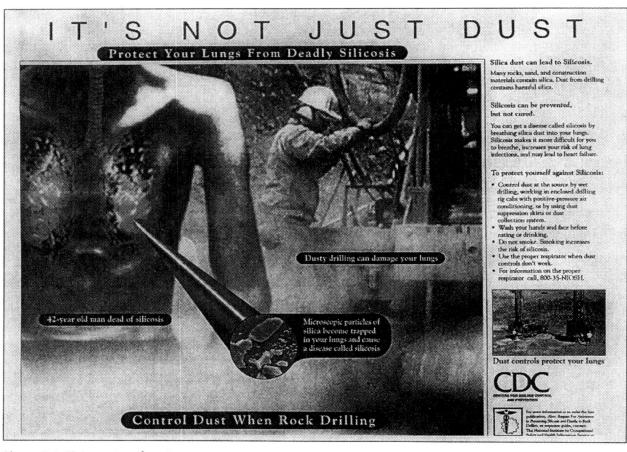

Figure 2.4 "It's not just dust."

WORKSHEET 4: UNDERSTANDING
HEALTH RISK MESSAGE CONCEPTS

The Threat Component
of a Health Risk Message

Name: _____

Date: _____

Course: _____

Section: _____

Professor: _____

Due: _____

■■
■■

Instructions: On the facing page is a health risk message. Please examine it carefully and answer the following questions completely. When asked to explain your answer, give reasons describing why you answered the question the way you did.

■■
■■

1. What is the threat in this health risk message?

   _____

   _____

   _____

2. What is the probability this threat will occur according to this message? Please explain. (*susceptibility to threat*)

   _____

   _____

   _____

3. Does this message make you feel susceptible to the threat? Why or why not? (*perceived susceptibility to threat*)

   _____

   _____

   _____

4. How noxious or unpleasant is the threat? Please explain. (*severity of threat*)

   _____

   _____

   _____

5. Does this message make you feel the threat is serious or trivial? Why or why not? (*perceived severity of threat*)

   _____

   _____

   _____

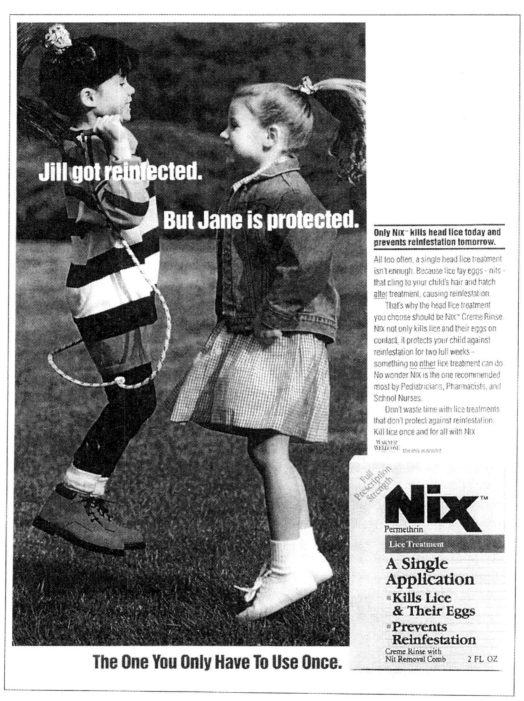

Figure 2.5 "Jill got reinfected . . ."

SOURCE: Reproduced with permission of Glaxo Wellcome, Inc. NIX is now owned by Warner-Lambert, a Pfizer Company.

WORKSHEET 5: UNDERSTANDING
HEALTH RISK MESSAGE CONCEPTS

The Efficacy Component
of a Health Risk Message

Name: _____

Date: _____

Course: _____

Section: _____

Due:_____

Professor: _____

Instructions: On the facing page is a health risk message. Please examine it carefully and answer the following questions completely. When asked to explain your answer, give reasons describing why you answered the question the way you did.

1. What is the recommended response in this health risk message?

_____

_____

_____

2. How effective is this recommended response in averting the threat, according to this message? Please explain. (*response efficacy*)

_____

_____

_____

3. Does this message make you feel the recommended response is effective in averting the threat? Why or why not? (*perceived response efficacy*)

_____

_____

_____

4. How easy or difficult is it to perform this recommended response, according to the message? Does the message indicate how to overcome any barriers to performing the recommended response? Please explain. (*self-efficacy*)

_____

_____

_____

5. Does this message make you feel able to perform the recommended response? Why or why not? (*perceived self-efficacy*)

_____

_____

_____

WORKSHEET 6: UNDERSTANDING THE EXTENDED PARALLEL PROCESS MODEL

Developing a Flow Chart
of People's Responses
According to the EPPM

Due:_____

Name: _____
Date: _____
Course: _____
Section: _____
Professor: _____

Instructions: Below is a blank flow chart. Fill in the correct terms and arrows according to the Extended Parallel Process Model. Give examples of what people's thoughts or responses might be where asked. Refer to Figure 3.1 and the text if you need help.

Hint: Words in the Flow Chart include fear control, danger control, fear, high perceived threat, low perceived threat, high perceived efficacy, low perceived efficacy, defensive motivation, protection motivation, no response, risk message. There should be 11 arrows.

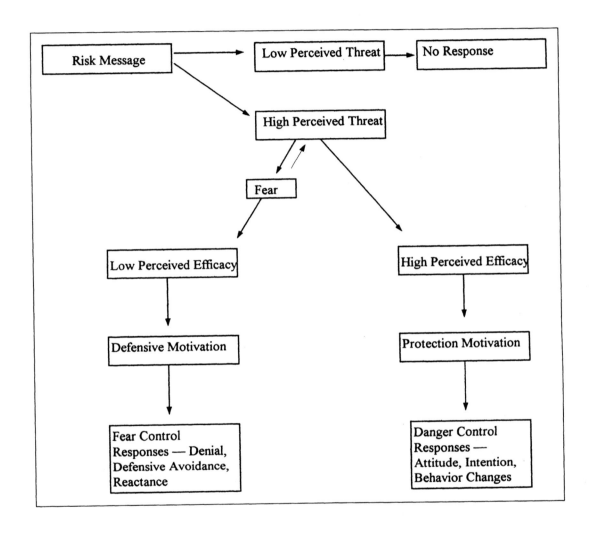

WORKSHEET 7: UNDERSTANDING THE EXTENDED PARALLEL PROCESS MODEL

Identifying Responses
According to the EPPM

Name: _____

Date: _____

Course: _____

Section: _____

Due:_____   Professor: _____

CHAPTER 3
WORKSHEETS

■■
■■

Instructions: Following are four distinct responses people gave to a risk message. Identify what level of perceived threat and perceived efficacy each person had and then indicate whether this person engaged in no response to the message, a danger control response, or a fear control response. Fully explain why you think this person engaged in a certain response.

■■
■■

Barbara, age 19, has had eight sexual partners in the last year.

I just like sex. I'm sorry but that's the way I am. And, I don't like just one partner—they get predictable so fast. But I'm not stupid either. I got chlamydia the very first time I had sex (I was 15). So I know that sexually transmitted diseases are real and I sure don't want to get any more—especially AIDS; that's a disease that really scares me. I knew someone who died from it and he wasted away to nothing. His thigh was as skinny as my forearm. That's why I always use condoms. I always have them with me and I use them as part of foreplay. It's easy to make them a fun part of sex. I know they work because I've never had a sexually transmitted disease since that first time. I get them for free at the campus health center.

a. Level of perceived threat (*severity and susceptibility*) Explain: _____

_____

b. Level of perceived efficacy (*self-efficacy and response efficacy*) Explain: _____

_____

c. Which response is Barbara engaging in? Why? _____

_____

■■
■■

Jack, age 47, has been a heavy smoker (2 packs a day) since age 20.

I've been smoking for almost 30 years and I enjoy it. I try quitting every five years or so but I guess my willpower's too weak. I start craving the smooth feeling and get antsy and downright cantankerous without cigarettes. I think my wife's actually relieved when I start up again. I've heard all of the hype about cigarettes causing lung cancer but you can't believe everything you read. My grandpa lived to 84 and he smoked half his life. All of those smoking studies are on rats anyway. Who's the government trying to kid?

a. Level of perceived threat (*severity and susceptibility*) Explain: _____

_____

b. Level of perceived efficacy (*self-efficacy and response efficacy*) Explain: _____

_____

c. Which response is Jack engaging in? Explain: _____

_____

▦

Aaron, age 29, rides a bike eight miles each day to and from work.

I never used to wear a bike helmet until one day my girlfriend and I were riding along a quiet country road. A car was going past us so we started to ride single file with her in front. She hit a rock just right with her tire and flipped head over on the bike. She skidded on her head a good three feet before she stopped. There was blood everywhere and a huge gash in the side of her head. She was unconscious by the time I reached her. I've never been more scared in my life. The car stopped and took us to the hospital where she had 39 stitches and was treated for shock. If she'd been wearing a helmet she would have been fine. Now I wear a helmet every time I ride my bike because I know they work. It's such an easy thing to do, too. I wish we had always done it.

a. Level of perceived threat (*severity and susceptibility*) Explain: _____

_____

b. Level of perceived efficacy (*self-efficacy and response efficacy*) Explain: _____

_____

c. Which response is Aaron engaging in? Why? _____

_____

▦

Lisa, age 30, does not wear seatbelt.

I've been driving since I was 15 years old and never been in a car accident. I don't even know anyone who's been in a car accident. I hate wearing seatbelts. They're so uncomfortable for short people like me. They cut into my neck. Besides, I'm a very safe driver, so I don't really need one."

a. Level of perceived threat (*severity and susceptibility*) Explain: _____

_____

b. Level of perceived efficacy (*self-efficacy and response efficacy*) Explain: _____

_____

c. Which response is Lisa engaging in? Why? _____

_____

WORKSHEET 8: APPLYING HEALTH BEHAVIOR CHANGE THEORIES

The Theory of Reasoned   Name: _____
Action: Gathering Salient   Date: _____
Beliefs and Salient Referents Course: _____
                              Section: _____
Due:_____   Professor: _____

■■
■■

Instructions: Choose a health issue and a target population. Ask representatives from your target population these questions to determine salient beliefs and referents.

■■
■■

1. What is your health threat? (be specific) _____

    _____

2. What are your recommended responses to avert the health threat? _____

    _____

According to the Theory of Reasoned Action, you must determine salient beliefs with regard to your "attitude object," which is your specific recommended response(s). To determine salient beliefs and referents, ask the following questions:

1. What are the advantages to [*doing recommended response*]?

    _____

    _____

    _____

2. What are the disadvantages to [*doing recommended response*]?

    _____

    _____

    _____

3. What people or groups of people might influence whether you [*do recommended response*]?

    _____

    _____

    _____

WORKSHEET 9: APPLYING HEALTH BEHAVIOR CHANGE THEORIES

Determining Attitudes
Toward the Recommended
Response According to
Theory of Reasoned Action
Due:_____

Name: _____
Date: _____
Course: _____
Section: _____
Professor: _____

⊞

Instructions: List the beliefs gathered in Worksheet 8 below (see Worksheet 8, items 1 and 2) and find out the strengths of their belief and the evaluations of that belief. Assess this information with different members of your target population. Determine their attitude toward your recommended response. Generate campaign messages.

⊞

Belief 1: _____

a. Indicate the degree to which you agree with this statement.

1	2	3	4	5	6	7
Not at all			Neutral			Totally True

b. Indicate whether you believe this statement is:

-3	-2	-1	0	+1	+2	+3
Bad						Good

Belief 2: _____

a. Indicate the degree to which you agree with this statement.

1	2	3	4	5	6	7
Not at all			Neutral			Totally True

b. Indicate whether or not you believe this statement is:

-3	-2	-1	0	+1	+2	+3
Bad						Good

Belief 3: _____

a. Indicate the degree to which you agree with this statement.

1	2	3	4	5	6	7
Not at all			Neutral			Totally True

b. Indicate whether or not you believe this statement is:

-3	-2	-1	0	+1	+2	+3
Bad						Good

Belief 4: _____

  a. Indicate the degree to which you agree with this statement.

1	2	3	4	5	6	7
Not at all			Neutral			Totally True

  b. Indicate whether or not you believe this statement is:

-3	-2	-1	0	+1	+2	+3
Bad						Good

Belief 5: _____

  a. Indicate the degree to which you agree with this statement.

1	2	3	4	5	6	7
Not at all			Neutral			Totally True

  b. Indicate whether or not you believe this statement is:

-3	-2	-1	0	+1	+2	+3
Bad						Good

Put this information into the following table, multiply strength of belief by evaluation of that belief, and sum the products to determine the overall attitude toward your recommended response. See Table 4.1 in Chapter 4 for help.

Attitude Toward _____ (*fill in your recommended response*)

Salient Beliefs	Strength of Beliefs (#a)	Evaluation of Beliefs(#b)	Product
1.			
2.			
3.			
4.			
5.			

Total Attitude Toward _____ (sum):_____ (*your recommended response*)

1. Is the overall attitude toward your recommended response positive or negative? (*explain*)

_____

_____

2. Develop some campaign messages to shift these beliefs (be creative). How do these messages address the beliefs, belief strengths, and evaluations of those beliefs (*explain*)?

1. _____

2. _____

3. _____

4. _____

5. _____

WORKSHEET 10: QUESTIONS FOR
THE HEALTH RISK MESSAGE DEVELOPER

Due: _____

Name: _____
Date: _____
Course: _____
Section: _____
Professor: _____

1. What threat are you trying to prevent? _____

_____

_____

_____

2. What is the recommended response to avert the threat, that is, the specific objective of the campaign?

_____

_____

_____

3. Who is the target audience (be specific; define the target population according to demographic variables, for example, socioeconomic status, literacy level, age, employment, residence, primary language, and so on; psychographic variables, for example, beliefs, values, worldview; and culture, for example, customs, and norms)? _____

_____

_____

_____

WORKSHEET 11: OPEN-ENDED QUESTIONS TO DETERMINE SALIENT BELIEFS ABOUT THE THREAT, APPROPRIATE RECOMMENDED RESPONSES, AND SALIENT REFERENTS

Due: _____

Name: _____

Date: _____

Course: _____

Section: _____

Professor: _____

1. What are your beliefs about [performing the recommended response]? *(attitude toward recommended response)* _____

_____

_____

_____

2. What negative consequences, if any, come from not [performing the recommended response]? *(determines audience perceptions of the threat)* _____

_____

_____

_____

3. What is the best way to prevent experiencing the negative consequences just identified? *(determines audience perceptions of the "best" recommended response)* _____

_____

_____

_____

4. Please list the people or groups who have an important influence on your [using the recommended response]. *(salient referents for subjective norm)* _____

_____

_____

_____

WORKSHEET 12: OPEN-ENDED QUESTIONS
TO DETERMINE SALIENT BELIEFS ABOUT
THREAT, EFFICACY, AND BENEFITS/BARRIERS

Due: _____

Name: _____

Date: _____

Course: _____

Section: _____

Professor: _____

1. How serious is [threat/negative consequences]? Please explain. *(perceived severity of the threat)*

_____

_____

2. How likely is it you will experience the [threat/negative consequences] if you do not [perform the recommended response]? Please explain. *(determines perceived susceptibility to the threat)*

_____

_____

3. Do you believe the [recommended response] prevents you from experiencing the [threat/negative consequences]? Why or why not? *(determines perceived response efficacy)*

_____

_____

4. Do you believe you can easily perform the [recommended response] to prevent yourself from experiencing the [threat/negative consequences]? Why or why not? *(determines perceived self-efficacy)*

_____

_____

5. What might keep you from performing the [recommended response]? Please explain. *(determines perceived barriers)*

_____

_____

6. What benefits do you perceive from performing the [recommended response]? Please explain. *(determines perceived benefits)*

_____

_____

WORKSHEET 13: CLOSED-ENDED QUESTIONS TO DETERMINE PERCEPTIONS OF THE THREAT AND RECOMMENDED RESPONSE

Due: _____

Name: _____

Date: _____

Course: _____

Section: _____

Professor: _____

1. I am at risk for [experiencing the threat]. *(perceived susceptibility)*

1	2	3	4	5	6	7
Strongly Disagree						Strongly Agree

2. [The threat] is serious. *(perceived severity)*

1	2	3	4	5	6	7
Strongly Disagree						Strongly Agree

3. [Performing the recommended response] will prevent [the threat]. *(perceived response efficacy)*

1	2	3	4	5	6	7
Strongly Disagree						Strongly Agree

4. I am easily able to [perform the recommended response]. *(perceived self-efficacy)*

1	2	3	4	5	6	7
Strongly Disagree						Strongly Agree

WORKSHEET 14: DETERMINING MORE AUDIENCE VARIABLES

Due: _____

Name: _____

Date: _____

Course: _____

Section: _____

Professor: _____

1. Please rank order the ways you prefer to learn about the [recommended response], with "1" representing your most preferred way of learning about the recommended response and "7" representing your least preferred way. *(preferred channel)*

   _____ television _____ magazine _____ newspaper _____ Internet _____ radio

   _____ interpersonal (face-to-face) channel _____ other (specify) _____

2. Please rank order from the person you would believe the most to the person you would believe the least if you received a message from him or her regarding [recommended response]. The numeral "1" represents the source you'd believe the most and "7" represents the source you'd believe the least. *(preferred source)*

   _____ health care professional _____ celebrity _____ Surgeon General _____ my parents

   _____ my colleagues _____ my friends _____ others (specify) _____

3. Please rank order the type of message you'd like to receive most for this [recommended response]. The numeral "1" represents your most preferred message type and "8" represents your least preferred message type.

   _____ message with lots of facts _____ entertaining message _____ comic-type message

   _____ message using stories of real people's experiences _____ message with good arguments

   _____ message that influences me emotionally _____ scary message

   _____ other type of message:_____

4. Respond "yes" or "no" to each of the following statements concerning your thoughts and actions. *(stage of change)*

   a. _____ Yes _____ No I have thought about [doing the recommended response]. *(precontemplation)*

   b. _____ Yes _____ No I have thought about [doing recommended response], but have not taken any steps to [do it] yet. *(contemplation)*

   c. _____ Yes _____ No I have not yet [done recommended response], but have taken steps so that I can soon (give examples). *(preparation—never used)*

   d. _____ Yes _____ No I have [done recommended response]. *(action)*

   e. _____ Yes _____ No I regularly [do recommended response]. *(maintenance)*

   f. _____ Yes _____ No I have [done recommended response] before, but currently do not [do it]. *(relapse; go to either preparation or contemplation stage)*

WORKSHEET 15: CONDUCTING FORMATIVE RESEARCH

Collecting Data from
a Target Audience

Name: _____

Date: _____

Course: _____

Section: _____

Due:_____   Professor: _____

■■
■■

Instructions: Following are the five steps to conducting formative research in preparation for developing your message. First, identify your threat and recommended response and describe your specific target audience (Step 1). Then, survey or interview at least one member of your target audience (Steps 2 to 5). Use classmates if necessary.

■■
■■

Step 1.   Goals and Objectives—Questions for Health Risk Message Developer:

1. What is the threat or negative consequence you are trying to prevent? _____

2. What is the recommended response to avert the threat or negative consequence *(the specific objective of the campaign)*? _____

3. Who is the target audience (be specific)? _____

Define target population according to demographic variables (e.g., socio-economic status, literacy level, age, employment, residence, primary language, etc.), psychographic variables (e.g., beliefs, values, worldview), and culture (e.g., customs, norms).

Step 2.   Open-Ended Questions to Determine Salient Beliefs about the Threat, Appropriate Recommended Responses, and Salient Referents

1. What are your beliefs about [performing recommended response]? *(determines attitude toward recommended response)*

_____

2. What negative consequences, if any, come from not [performing recommended response]? *(determines audience perceptions of the threat)*

_____

3. What is the best way to prevent experiencing the negative consequences just identified? *(determines audience perceptions of the best recommended response)*

_____

4. Please list the people or groups who have an important influence on your [using recommended response]? *(determines salient referents for subjective norm)*

_____

Step 3. Open-Ended Questions to Determine Salient Beliefs about Theoretical Variables

1. How serious is [negative consequence/threat]? Please explain. *(determines perceived severity of the threat).*

   _____

2. How likely is it that you will experience the [negative consequence/threat] because you do not [perform the recommended response]? Please explain. *(determines perceived susceptibility to the threat)*

   _____

3. [Recommended response] will keep me from experiencing the [negative consequence/threat]. Why or why not? *(determines perceived response efficacy)*

   _____

4. I can easily do the [recommended response] to prevent my experiencing the [negative consequence/threat]. Why or why not? *(determines perceived self-efficacy)*

   _____

5. What keeps you from performing the [recommended reponse]? Please explain. *(determines perceived barriers)*

   _____

6. What benefits do you see from performing the [recommended response]? Please explain. *(determines perceived benefits)*

   _____

Step 4. Closed-Ended Questions to Determine Threat and Recommended Response Perceptions

1. I am at risk for [experiencing threat]. *(determines perceived susceptibility)*

1	2	3	4	5	6	7
Strongly Disagree						Strongly Agree

2. [The threat] is serious. *(determines perceived severity)*

1	2	3	4	5	6	7
Strongly Disagree						Strongly Agree

3. [Doing recommended response] prevents [the threat]. *(determines perceived response efficacy)*

1	2	3	4	5	6	7
Strongly Disagree						Strongly Agree

4. I am easily able to [do recommended response]. *(determines perceived self-efficacy)*

1	2	3	4	5	6	7
Strongly Disagree						Strongly Agree

Step 5. Additional Audience Variables to Determine

1. Please place in rank order the ways you prefer to learn about the [recommended response], with "1" representing your most preferred way of learning about the recommended response and "7" representing your least favored way of learning about the recommended response. *(determines preferred channel)*

   _____ television _____ magazine _____ letter from professional organization _____ radio

   _____ colleague _____ my boss _____ other (specify): _____

2. Please place in rank order the person you would believe the most to the person you would believe the least if you received a message about the [recommended response] from him or her, with "1" representing the most believable person and "7" representing the least believable person? *(determines preferred source)*

   _____ health care professional _____ library expert _____ Surgeon General _____ the AMA

   _____ my boss _____ my colleagues _____ other (specify): _____

3. Please place in rank order the type of message you'd like to receive most for this [recommended response], with "1" representing your most preferred message type and "8" representing your least preferred message type.

   _____ message with lots of facts _____ entertaining message _____ comic-type message

   _____ message using stories of real people's experience _____ message with good arguments

   _____ message that influences me emotionally _____ scary message

   _____ other type of message:_____

4. Choose the response that best represents your thoughts and actions: *(determines stage of change)*

   a. _____ Yes _____ No   I have yet to think about [doing recommended response]. *(determines precontemplation)*

   b. _____ Yes _____ No   I have thought about [doing recommended response] but have not taken any steps to [do it] yet. *(determines contemplation)*

   c. _____ Yes _____ No   I have not yet [done recommended response] but have taken steps so I can do so soon (e.g., give examples). *(determines preparation—never used)*

   d. _____ Yes _____ No   I have [done recommended response]. *(determines action)*

   e. _____ Yes _____ No   I regularly [do recommended response]. *(determines maintenance)*

   f. _____ Yes _____ No   I have [done recommended response] before, but currently do not [do it]. *(determines relapse; go to either preparation or contemplation stage)*

WORKSHEET 16: THE RISK BEHAVIOR DIAGNOSIS SCALE

Understanding the Concepts

Name: _____

Date: _____

Course: _____

Section: _____

Due:_____   Professor: _____

■■
■■

Instructions: To use the RBD Scale quickly, you need a very clear understanding of each construct. The following are several variations of statements from the Risk Behavior Diagnosis Scale across different topics. Match each statement with its appropriate construct. In the far right column, indicate whether the statement represents susceptibility (SUSC), severity (SEV), response efficacy (RE) or self-efficacy (SE).

■■
■■

Susceptibility = SUSC   Severity = SEV   Response Efficacy = RE   Self-Efficacy = SE

1. I will not get AIDS if I use a condom.   _____
2. I can use condoms each time I have sex   _____
3. Skin cancer is harmful.   _____
4. I am susceptible to being injured in a drunk driving accident.   _____
5. I am able to exercise 30 minutes or more three times a week.   _____
6. Osteoporosis is a serious health threat.   _____
7. It is possible that I will be harmed by environmental pollutants.   _____
8. Breast self-examinations are effective in preventing my dying
    from breast cancer.   _____
9. It is easy to use sun screen every time I'm in the sun.   _____
10. Bike helmets prevent injuries from bike accidents.   _____
11. I am at risk for getting colon cancer.   _____
12. Most car accidents cause serious injuries.   _____
13. I am able to do breast self-examinations.   _____
14. It is easy to wear a bicycle helmet every time I ride my bike.   _____
15. It is likely that I will suffer a heart attack.   _____
16. Injuries from bike accidents are harmful.   _____
17. Hepatitis is a severe health threat.   _____
18. Eating four vegetables a day prevents cancers of all kinds.   _____
19. It is easy for me to get a flu shot.   _____
20. Washing my hands prevents transmission of cold viruses.   _____
21. Tuberculosis is a serious health threat.   _____
22. I will not get HIV if I use condoms.   _____
23. I am at risk for getting breast cancer.   _____
24. I am likely to be in a serious car accident in my life.   _____

Assessing Your Own
Client with the RBD Scale"

Name: _____

Date: _____

Course: _____

Section: _____

Due: _____

Professor: _____

Instructions: The following is a case study of a client who presented for HIV counseling and testing. Assess the RBD Scale. Determine if the client is in fear control, danger control, or has low threat perceptions. Offer your recommendations on developing an effective health risk message.

Risk and Background Information

Jack is a 21-year-old heterosexual male. His risk is unprotected vaginal intercourse with several women. He has moderate anxiety and states he uses condoms on occasion. He uses alcohol when he engages in sex.

	Strongly Disagree				Strongly Agree	
1. Using condoms is effective in preventing AIDS.	1	2	3	④	5	
2. Condoms work in preventing AIDS.	1	2	3	④	5	ΣRE =
3. If I use a condom, I am less likely to get AIDS.	1	2	3	4	⑤	
4. Using condoms to prevent AIDS is convenient.	1	2	③	4	5	
5. Using condoms to prevent AIDS is easy.	1	2	3	④	5	ΣSE =
6. I am able to use condoms to prevent getting AIDS.	1	2	3	④	5	
						ΣEFFICACY =
7. I believe that AIDS is severe.	1	2	3	4	⑤	
8. I believe AIDS is a significant disease.	1	2	3	4	⑤	ΣSEV =
9. I believe that AIDS is serious.	1	2	3	4	⑤	
10. It is likely that I will contract AIDS	1	②	3	4	5	
11. I am at risk for getting AIDS	1	②	3	4	5	ΣSUSC =
12. It is possible that I will contract AIDS	1	②	3	4	5	
						ΣTHREAT =

DISCRIMINATING VALUE =

Legend: Σ = Sum of; RE = Response; SE = Self-Efficacy; SEV = Severity; SUSC = Susceptibility.

Jack is engaging in: (circle one)   Danger Control   Fear Control   Low Threat Perception

Based on the scores for the four individual divisions (response efficacy, self-efficacy, severity of threat, and susceptibility to threat), which, if any, additional questions would you ask?

_____

_____

_____

_____

_____

Describe the most effective type of health risk message for this person. Explain why you believe this type of message would be effective for this person.

_____

_____

_____

_____

_____

_____

WORKSHEET 18: CASE SIX—
RISK BEHAVIOR DIAGNOSIS SCALE

Assessing Your Own
Client with the RBD Scale

Name: _____

Date: _____

Course: _____

Section: _____

Due:_____ Professor: _____

██
██

Instructions: The following is a case study of a client who presented for HIV counseling and testing. Assess the RBD Scale. Determine whether the client is in fear control, danger control, or has low threat perceptions. Offer your recommendations on how to develop an effective health risk message.

██
██

Risk and Background Information

Emily is an 18-year-old heterosexual female. Her risk is unprotected vaginal and oral intercourse with several men. She has extreme anxiety and states she does not like to use condoms. She always uses alcohol when she has sex.

██
██

	Strongly Disagree				Strongly Agree	
1. Using condoms is effective in preventing AIDS.	1	2	3	④	5	
2. Condoms work in preventing AIDS.	1	2	3	④	5	ΣRE =
3. If I use a condom, I am less likely to get AIDS.	1	2	3	4	⑤	
4. Using condoms to prevent AIDS is convenient.	1	2	③	4	5	
5. Using condoms to prevent AIDS is easy.	1	2	3	④	5	ΣSE =
6. I am able to use condoms to prevent getting AIDS.	1	2	3	④	5	
						ΣEFFICACY =
7. I believe that AIDS is severe.	1	2	3	4	⑤	
8. I believe AIDS is a significant disease.	1	2	3	4	⑤	ΣSEV =
9. I believe that AIDS is serious.	1	2	3	4	⑤	
10. It is likely that I will contract AIDS	1	②	3	4	5	
11. I am at risk for getting AIDS	1	②	3	4	5	ΣSUSC =
12. It is possible that I will contract AIDS	1	②	3	4	5	
						ΣTHREAT =

DISCRIMINATING VALUE =

Legend: Σ = Sum of; RE = Response; SE = Self-Efficacy; SEV = Severity; SUSC = Susceptibility.

Emily is engaging in: (circle one)   Danger Control   Fear Control   Low Threat Perception

Based on the scores for the four individual divisions (response efficacy, self-efficacy, severity of threat, and susceptibility to threat), which, if any, additional questions would you ask?

_____

_____

_____

_____

_____

_____

Describe the most effective type of health risk message for this person. Explain why you believe this type of message would be effective for this person.

_____

_____

_____

_____

_____

_____

WORKSHEET 19: CASE SEVEN—
RISK BEHAVIOR DIAGNOSIS SCALE

Assessing Your Own Client   Name: _____
with the RBD Scale   Date: _____
                                     Course: _____
                                     Section: _____
Due:_____   Professor: _____

■■
■■

Instructions: The following is a case study of a client who presented for HIV counseling and testing. Assess the RBD Scale. Determine whether the client is in fear control, danger control, or has low threat perceptions. Offer your recommendations on how to develop an effective health risk message.

■■
■■

Risk and Background Information

Taylor is a 19-year-old gay male. His risk is unprotected anal and oral intercourse (some receptive) with several men. He has low to moderate anxiety and states he does not use condoms because he knows his partners are not risky. He uses alcohol only on occasion.

■■
■■

	Strongly Disagree				Strongly Agree	
1. Using condoms is effective in preventing AIDS.	1	2	3	④	5	
2. Condoms work in preventing AIDS.	1	2	3	④	5	ΣRE =
3. If I use a condom, I am less likely to get AIDS.	1	2	3	4	⑤	
4. Using condoms to prevent AIDS is convenient.	1	2	3	4	⑤	
5. Using condoms to prevent AIDS is easy.	1	2	3	④	5	ΣSE =
6. I am able to use condoms to prevent getting AIDS.	1	2	3	4	⑤	
						ΣEFFICACY =
7. I believe that AIDS is severe.	1	2	3	4	⑤	
8. I believe AIDS is a significant disease.	1	2	3	4	⑤	ΣSEV =
9. I believe that AIDS is serious.	1	2	3	4	⑤	
10. It is likely that I will contract AIDS	①	2	3	4	5	
11. I am at risk for getting AIDS	1	2	③	4	5	ΣSUSC =
12. It is possible that I will contract AIDS	1	②	3	4	5	
						ΣTHREAT =

DISCRIMINATING VALUE =

Legend: Σ = Sum of; RE = Response; SE = Self-Efficacy; SEV = Severity; SUSC = Susceptibility.

Taylor is engaging in: (circle one)   Danger Control   Fear Control   Low Threat Perception

Based on the scores for the four individual divisions (response efficacy, self-efficacy, severity of threat, and susceptibility to threat), which, if any, additional questions would you ask?

_____

_____

_____

_____

_____

_____

Describe the most effective type of health risk message for this person. Explain why you believe this type of message would be effective for this person.

_____

_____

_____

_____

_____

_____

WORKSHEET 20: THE RISK BEHAVIOR DIAGNOSIS SCALE

Developing Your Own RBD Scale

Name: _____

Date: _____

Course: _____

Section: _____

Due:_____

Professor: _____

∷

Instructions: The following is a template for the Risk Behavior Diagnosis Scale. Develop your own scale and administer it to three people. Determine whether each person is in fear control, danger control, or has low threat perceptions. Offer your recommendations on how to develop an effective health risk message. Use classmates if necessary.

∷

1. What is your health threat? _____

2. What is your recommended response? _____

3. Fill in your health threat and recommended response in the appropriate places.

   a. I am able to _____

   b. It is easy to _____

   c. I can _____

   d. _____ prevents _____

   e. I will not get _____ if I _____

   f. _____ is effective in getting rid of _____

   g. I am at risk for _____

   h. It is possible that I will _____

   i. I am susceptible to _____

   j. _____ is a serious threat.

   k. _____ is harmful.

   l. _____ is a severe threat.

1. Ask three people to indicate their agreement or disagreement with each of these statements on a scale from "1"—strongly disagree to "7"—strongly agree.

1	2	3	4	5	6	7
Strongly Disagree						Strongly Agree

2. Add up each person's threat and efficacy scores. Subtract their threat score from their efficacy score. This is the discriminating value score. (Remember, Σ means "sum of," so simply add everything up.)

	Total Efficacy Score (Σ Perceived Efficacy)	Total Threat Score (Σ Perceived Threat)	Efficacy–Threat Score (Discriminating Value Score)
Person 1	_____	_____	_____
Person 2	_____	_____	_____
Person 3	_____	_____	_____

3. Now you have a discriminating value score for each person. Place each person into the following categories. You can list each person more than once.

Danger Control (positive discriminating value): _____

Fear Control (negative discriminating value): _____

Low Threat Perceptions (threat score < 12): _____

Low Response Efficacy Perceptions (Σd-f < 6): _____

Low Self-Efficacy Perceptions (Σa-c < 6): _____

Low Susceptibility Perceptions (Σg-i < 6): _____

Low Severity Perceptions (Σj-l < 6): _____

4. Describe the most effective type of health risk message for each person. Explain why you believe this type of health risk message is effective for this person.

Person 1 _____

_____

Person 2 _____

_____

Person 3 _____

_____

WORKSHEET 21: PROGRAM EVALUATION

Formative, Process, and
Outcome Evaluation

Name: _____

Date: _____

Course: _____

Section: _____

Due:_____

Professor: _____

Instructions: Imagine you are a student at a university where everyone goes to warm-weather places during Spring Break, which occurs the first week in March. In the past, students have sunburned themselves very badly attempting to tan, some even requiring hospitalization. To prevent this from happening this year, assume you have developed a campaign titled *Lay It On Me*, focused on reducing the incidence of sun poisoning among your classmates. This campaign is to occur during the last week in February. The goal and objectives are specified below. Furthermore, assume you have identified the following three activities to help you meet your short-term objectives: (1) hang posters in the school classrooms, (2) use peer-educators to conduct a series of workshops for students, and (3) distribute "buy one, get one free" coupons for sunscreen.

Short-term objectives	Long-term objective	Goal
Increase to 90% the number of students who feel susceptible to sun poisoning by March 1		
Increase to 90% the number of students who believe sun poisoning has severe consequences by March 1	Increase to 90% the number of students who use sunscreen (with the recommended SPF) each time they lay on the beach during Spring Break	Reduce the incidence of sun poisoning among students while on Spring Break
Increase to 90% the number of students who believe sun poisoning can be averted by consistently applying proper sunscreen by March 1		
Increase to 90% the number of students who believe they can consistently apply proper sunscreen by March 1		

1. Answer each of the following questions assuming you conduct formative evaluation research for this campaign.

   a. What is the purpose of your formative evaluation?

   _____

   _____

   _____

   _____

   b. When will you conduct your formative evaluation?

   _____

   c. Specifically describe the formative evaluation activities you engage in and provide a rationale for their inclusion. Be sure to include at least one preproduction and one postproduction formative activity.

   _____

   _____

   _____

   _____

   _____

   _____

   _____

   _____

2. Answer each of the following questions assuming you conduct a process evaluation for this campaign.

   a. What is the purpose of your process evaluation?

   _____

   _____

   _____

   _____

   b. When will you conduct your process evaluation?

   _____

   c. Specifically describe the process evaluation activities you engage in and provide a rationale for their inclusion.

   _____

   _____

   _____

   _____

   _____

   _____

   _____

3. Answer each of the following questions assuming you will conduct an outcome evaluation for this campaign.

    a. What is the purpose of your outcome evaluation?

_____

_____

_____

_____

    b. When will you conduct your outcome evaluation?

_____

    c. Specifically describe the outcome evaluation activities you engage in and provide a rationale for their inclusion. Be sure to discuss the research design you would use for your evaluation.

_____

_____

_____

_____

_____

_____

_____

WORKSHEET 22: FOCUS GROUPS

Developing a Focus Group Protocol

Name: _____
Date: _____
Course: _____
Section: _____
Professor: _____

Due:_____

⚏

Instructions: Assume your supervisor at the state health department has asked you to oversee a health communication campaign focused on motorcycle safety. Although you believe you have the skills necessary to do so, your knowledge of the topic is limited. Therefore, you decide it would be advantageous to conduct a focus group to learn more about the topic. Please respond to the following questions given this scenario.

⚏

1. Who would you invite to participate in the focus group? How many people would you invite and what would you do to make sure they attended?

_____
_____
_____
_____

2. Identify three main topics or knowledge areas you would emphasize during the focus group.

Topic 1 _____

Topic 2 _____

Topic 3 _____

3. For each topic identified above, develop three questions you would ask focus group members.

Topic 1

Question 1 _____
_____

Question 2 _____
_____

Question 3 _____
_____

Topic 2

    Question 1 _____

    _____

    Question 2 _____

    _____

    Question 3 _____

    _____

Topic 3

    Question 1 _____

    _____

    Question 2 _____

    _____

    Question 3 _____

    _____

4. Describe the process you would use to analyze the information obtained in your focus group.

_____

_____

_____

_____

_____

_____

_____

_____

_____

_____

WORKSHEET 23: MEASURES OF CENTRAL TENDENCY

Computing Measures
of Central Tendency

Name: _____

Date: _____

Course: _____

Section: _____

Due:_____

Professor: _____

∷

Instructions: The following are data from two groups of individuals. Assume the data were obtained from individuals presented with the statement, "I believe HIV is a severe disease" and asked to respond using the following scale:

"Strongly agree (5), Agree (4), Neutral (3), Disagree (2)," and "Strongly Disagree (1)." For each data set, compute the mean, median, and mode and explain what each measure tells you about the group.

∷

Group 1	Group 2
5	1
3	3
4	3
5	1
1	2

Mean (Group 1) _____   Mean (Group 2) _____

Explanation of group means _____

_____

Median (Group 1) _____   Median (Group 2) _____

Explanation of group medians _____

_____

Mode (Group 1) _____   Mode (Group 2) _____

Explanation of group modes _____

_____

WORKSHEET 24: MEASURES OF DISPERSION

Computing Measures of Dispersion

Name: _____

Date: _____

Course: _____

Section: _____

Due:_____

Professor: _____

■■
■■

Instructions: The following are data from two groups of individuals (same as in Worksheet 23). Assume the data were obtained from individuals presented with the statement, "I believe HIV is a severe disease" and asked to respond using the following scale:

"Strongly agree (5), Agree (4), Neutral (3), Disagree (2)," and "Strongly Disagree (1)." For each data set, compute the range, variance, and standard deviation and explain what each measure tells you about the group.

■■
■■

Group 1	*Group 2*
5	1
3	3
4	3
5	1
1	2

Range (Group 1) _____

Range (Group 2) _____

Explanation of group ranges _____

_____

Variance (Group 1) _____

Variance (Group 2) _____

Explanation of group variances _____

_____

Standard deviation (Group 1)_____

Standard deviation (Group 2) _____

Explanation of group standard deviations: _____

_____

WORKSHEET 25: COMPUTATION OF THE *t* TEST

Computing the t *Test*

Name: _____

Date: _____

Course: _____

Section: _____

Due:_____

Professor: _____

■■

Instructions: The following are data for two groups of individuals (same as Worksheets 23 & 24). Assume the data were obtained from individuals presented with the statement, "I believe HIV is a severe disease" and asked to respond using the following scale:

"Strongly agree (5), Agree (4), Neutral (3), Disagree (2)," and "Strongly Disagree (1)." Begin by stating the null hypothesis and the research hypothesis and then determine whether the response difference is statistically significant by computing the *t* statistic (show your computation). Finally, explain the meaning of your *t* score.

■■

Null hypothesis _____

_____

Research hypothesis _____

_____

t _____

Explanation of *t* score _____

_____

_____

_____

_____

_____

Table 9.6 *t Distribution*

df	Level of Significance for One-Tailed Test					
	.05	.025	.01	.005	.001	.0005
	Level of Significance for Two-Tailed Test					
	.10	.05	.02	.01	.002	.001
1	6.314	12.706	31.820	63.657	318.309	636.619
2	2.920	4.303	6.965	9.925	22.327	31.599
3	2.353	3.182	4.541	5.841	10.215	12.924
4	2.132	2.776	3.747	4.604	7.173	8.610
5	2.015	2.571	3.365	4.032	5.893	6.869
6	1.943	2.447	3.143	3.707	5.208	5.959
7	1.895	2.365	2.998	3.499	4.785	5.408
8	1.860	2.306	2.896	3.355	4.501	5.041
9	1.833	2.262	2.821	3.250	4.297	4.781
10	1.812	2.228	2.764	3.169	4.144	4.587
11	1.796	2.201	2.718	3.106	4.025	4.437
12	1.782	2.179	2.681	3.055	3.930	4.318
13	1.771	2.160	2.650	3.012	3.852	4.221
14	1.761	2.145	2.624	2.977	3.787	4.140
15	1.753	2.131	2.602	2.947	3.733	4.073
16	1.746	2.120	2.583	2.921	3.686	4.015
17	1.740	2.110	2.567	2.898	3.646	3.965
18	1.734	2.101	2.552	2.878	3.610	3.922
19	1.729	2.093	2.539	2.861	3.579	3.883
20	1.725	2.086	2.528	2.845	3.552	3.850
21	1.721	2.080	2.518	2.831	3.527	3.819
22	1.717	2.074	2.508	2.819	3.505	3.792
23	1.714	2.069	2.500	2.807	3.485	3.768
24	1.711	2.064	2.492	2.797	3.467	3.745
25	1.708	2.060	2.485	2.787	3.450	3.725
26	1.706	2.056	2.479	2.779	3.435	3.707
27	1.703	2.052	2.473	2.771	3.421	3.690
28	1.701	2.048	2.467	2.763	3.408	3.674
29	1.699	2.045	3.462	2.756	3.396	3.659
30	1.697	2.042	2.457	2.750	3.385	3.646
50	1.676	2.009	2.403	2.678	3.261	3.496
100	1.660	1.984	2.364	2.626	3.174	3.390
∞	1.645	1.960	2.326	2.576	3.090	3.291

SOURCE: From Mary B. Harris, *Basic Statistics for Behavioral Science Research* (2nd ed.), p.157. Copyright © 1998 by Allyn & Bacon. Reprinted by permission.

WORKSHEET 26: GETTING THE MESSAGE OUT

Developing a Budget
for a Media Mix

Name: _____

Date: _____

Course: _____

Section: _____

Due:_____

Professor: _____

Instructions: Imagine you are in charge of a health communication campaign and you are trying to determine what media to use to get your message out. Call local media outlets to determine the cost of different media.

1. How much does a 30-second spot on a local television station cost?
   a. during prime time _____
   b. during the evening news _____
   c. between the hours of midnight and 4am _____
   d. during the afternoon hours _____

2. How much does a 30-second spot on your favorite local radio station cost?
   a. during morning drive-time _____
   b. between mid-morning and mid-afternoon _____
   c. during afternoon drive-time _____
   d. between the hours of midnight and 4am _____

3. How much does an advertisement in your local newspaper cost? (get costs for a variety of sizes)
   a. small _____
   b. medium _____
   c. large _____

4. How much does it cost to rent space on a billboard for:
   a. one month _____
   b. six months _____
   c. one year _____

5. What are the costs for printing the following (in three colors):

   a. Flyers   (100) _____   (1,000) _____   (10,000) _____
   b. Pamphlets   (100) _____   (1,000) _____   (10,000) _____
   c. Posters   (100) _____   (1,000) _____   (10,000)_____

WORKSHEET 27: FIELD APPLICATION

*Investigating an
Existing Health Campaign*

Name: _____
Date: _____
Course: _____
Section: _____

Due:_____

Professor: _____

◪

Instructions: Choose an existing ongoing mediated health campaign and answer the following questions as best you can.

◪

1. What is the threat or negative consequence they are trying to prevent?

   _____
   _____

2. What is the recommended response to avert the threat or negative consequence?

   _____
   _____

3. Who is the target audience for this campaign (be as specific as possible)?

   _____
   _____

4. What is the medium through which the message is delivered?

   _____
   _____

5. Do you believe this particular medium is preferred by target audience members? Explain.

   _____
   _____
   _____
   _____

6. Do you believe this message will be accessible to target audience members? Explain.

_____

_____

_____

_____

7. Who is the message source? How credible do you believe this source is for target audience members? Explain.

_____

_____

_____

_____

8. Overall, how effective do you think this campaign is? Explain.

_____

_____

_____

_____

9. What changes would you suggest be made to the presentation of the threat?

_____

_____

_____

_____

10. What changes would you suggest be made to the presentation of the recommended response?

_____

_____

_____

_____

References

Ajzen, I, & Fishbein, M. (1980). *Understanding attitudes and predicting social behavior.* Upper Saddle River, NJ: Prentice-Hall.

Alvaro, E. M., & Burgoon, M. (1995). Individual differences in responses to social influence attempts: Theory and research on the effects of misanthropy. *Communication Research, 22,* pp. 347-384.

Andersen, P. A., & Guerrero, L.K. (1998). *The handbook of communication and emotion: Research, theory, applications, and contexts.* San Diego, CA: Academic Press.

Atkin, C. K., & Freimuth, V. (1989). Formative evaluation research in campaign design. In R. E. Rice & C. K. Atkin (Eds.) *Public communication campaigns* (2nd ed., pp. 131-150). Newbury Park, CA: Sage.

Bandura, A. (1977). Self-efficacy: Toward a unifying theory of behavioral change. *Psychological Review, 84,* 191-215.

Bandura, A. (1989). Perceived self-efficacy in the exercise of control over AIDS infection. In V. M. Mays, G. W. Albee, and S. F. Schneider (Eds.), *Primary prevention of AIDS: Psychological approaches* (128-141). Newbury Park, CA: Sage.

Bang, H. K. (1993). *The effectiveness of the use of fear appeals depicting legal and physical consequences in anti-drunk driving television public service announcements.* Unpublished doctoral dissertation, Michigan State University.

Beck, K. H. (1979). The effects of positive and negative arousal upon attitudes, belief acceptance, behavioral intention, behavior. *The Journal of Social Psychology, 107,* 239-251.

Beck, K. H., & Davis, C. M. (1978). Effects of fear-arousing communications and topic importance on attitude change. *Journal of Social Psychology, 104,* 81-95.

Beck, K. H., & Frankel, A. (1981). A conceptualization of threat communications and protective health behavior. *Social Psychology Quarterly, 44,* 204-217.

Beck, K. H., & Lund, A. K. (1981). The effects of health threat seriousness and personal efficacy upon intentions and behavior. *Journal of Applied Social Psychology, 11,* 401-405.

Berkowitz, L., & Cottingham, D. R. (1960). The interest value and relevance of fear arousing communications. *Journal of Abnormal and Social Psychology, 1,* 37-43.

Boster, F. J., & Mongeau, P. (1984). Fear-arousing persuasive messages. In R. N. Bostrom & B. H. Westley (Eds.), *Communication yearbook 8* (pp. 330-375). Newbury Park, CA: Sage.

Brouwers, M. C., & Sorrentino, R. M. (1993). Uncertainty orientation and protection motivation theory: The role of individual differences in health compliance. *Journal of Personality and Social Psychology, 65,* 102-112.

Brubaker, R. G., & Wickersham, D. (1990). Encouraging the practice of testicular self-examination: A field application of the theory of reasoned action. *Health Psychology, 9,* 154-163.

Burgoon, M. (1989). Messages and persuasive effects. In J.J. Bradac (Ed.), *Message effects in communication science* (pp. 129-164). Newbury Park, CA: Sage.

Burnett, J. J. (1981). Internal-external locus of control as a moderator of fear appeals. *Journal of Applied Psychology, 66,* 390-393.

Burnett, J. J., & Oliver, R. L. (1979). Fear appeal effects in the field: A segmentation approach. *Journal of Marketing Research, 16,* 181-190.

Centers for Disease Control and Prevention (CDC) (1994). *HIV counseling, testing and referral standards & guidelines.* Washington, DC: U.S. Department of Health & Human Services, Public Health Service.

Chaiken, S. (1980). Heuristic versus systematic information processing and the use of source versus message cues in persuasion. *Journal of Personality and Social Psychology, 39,* 752-766.

Chaiken, S. (1987). The heuristic model of persuasion. In M. P. Zanna, J. M. Olson, & C. P. Herman (Eds.), *Social influence: The Ontario symposium* (Vol. 5, pp. 3-39). Hillsdale, NJ: Lawrence Erlbaum.

Chu, G. C. (1966). Fear arousal, efficacy, and imminency. *Journal of Personality and Social Psychology, 4,* 517-524.

Cohen, J. (1988). *Statistical power analysis for the behavioral sciences* (2nd ed.). Hillsdale, NJ: Lawrence Erlbaum.

Crawford, T. J., & Boyer, R. (1985). Salient consequences, cultural values, and childbearing intentions. *Journal of Applied Social Psychology, 15,* 16-30.

Crawford, T. J., & Leventhal, H. (1966). Effects of varying the recommendations in a fear-arousing communication. *Journal of Personality and Social Psychology, 4,* 525-531.

Dabbs, J. M. (1964). Self-esteem, communicator characteristics, and attitude change. *Journal of Abnormal and Social Psychology, 69,* 173-181.

Dabbs, J. M., & Leventhal, H. (1966). Effects of varying the recommendations of a fear-arousing communciation. *Journal of Personality and Social Psychology, 4,* 525-531.

Dearing, J. W., & Rogers, E. M. (1995). *Strategies of HIV prevention programs in San Francisco.* Paper presented at the Symposium on Communicating Health with Unique Population Groups, Michigan State University, April 8-9.

Dearing, J. W., Rogers, E. M., Meyer, G., Casey, M. K., Rao, N., Campo, S., & Henderson, G. M. (1996). Social marketing and diffusion-based strategies for communicating health with unique populations: HIV prevention in San Francisco. *Journal of Health Communication, 1,* 343-363.

Dembroski, T. M., Lasater, T. M., & Ramirez, A. (1978). Communicator similarity, fear arousing communications, and compliance with health care recommendations. *Journal of Applied Social Psychology, 8,* 254-269.

DiClemente, C. C., & Prochaska, J. O. (1985). Processes and stages of change: Coping and competence in smoking behavior change. In S. Shiffman & T. A. Willis (Eds.), *Coping and substance abuse* (pp. 319- 334). San Diego, CA: Academic Press.

Dillard, J. P. (1994). Rethinking the study of fear appeals: An emotional perspective. *Communication Theory, 4,* 295-323.

Dorfman, L. E., Derish, P. A., & Cohen, J. B. (1992). Hey girlfriend: An evaluation of AIDS prevention among women in the sex industry. *Health Education Quarterly, 19*(1), 25-40.

Eisen, M., Zellman, G. I., & McAllister, A. L. (1985). A health belief model approach to adolescents' fertility control: Some pilot program findings. *Health Education Quarterly, 12,* 185-210.

Ferguson, K. J., Yesalis, C. E., Pomrehn, P. R., & Kirkpatrick, M. B. (1989). Attitudes, knowledge, and beliefs as predictors of exercise intent and behavior in schoolchildren. *Journal of School Health, 59,* 112-115.

Fishbein, M., & Ajzen, I. (1975). *Belief, attitude, intention, and behavior: An introduction to theory and research.* Reading, MA: Addison-Wesley.

Fishbein, M., & Ajzen, I. (1981). Acceptance, yielding and impact: Cognitive processes in persuasion. In R.E. Petty, T.M. Ostrom, & T.C. Brock (Eds.), Cognitive responses in persuasion (pp. 339-359). Hillsdale, NJ: Lawrence Erlbaum.

Fishbein, M., Ajzen, I., & McArdle, J. (1980). Changing the behavior of alcoholics: Effects of persuasive communication. In I. Ajzen & M. Fishbein (Eds.), *Understanding attitudes and predicting social behavior.* Englewood Cliffs, NJ: Prentice-Hall.

Fishbein, M., & Middlestadt, S. E. (1989). Using the theory of reasoned action as a framework for understanding and changing AIDS-related behaviors. In V. M. Mays, G. W. Albee, & S. S. Schneider (Eds.), *Primary prevention of AIDS: Psychological approaches* (pp. 93-110). Newbury Park, CA: Sage.

Fishbein, M., Middlestadt, S. E., & Hitchcock, P. J. (1991). Using information to change sexually transmitted disease related behaviors: An analysis based on the theory of reasoned action. In J.N. Wasserheit, S.O. Aral, and K. K. Holmes (Eds.), *Research issues in human behavior change and sexually transmitted diseases in the AIDS era* (pp. 243-257). Washington DC: American Society for Microbiology.

Fletcher, J. L. (1991, January). Perinatal transmission of human papillomavirus. *American Family Physician,* January, 143-146.

Frandsen, K. D. (1963). Effects of threat appeals and media of transmission. *Speech Monographs, 30,* 101-104.

Frey, K. P., & Eagly, A. H. (1993). Vividness can undermine the persuasiveness of messages. *Journal of Personality and Social Psychology, 65,* 32-44.

Fritzen, R. D., & Mazer, G. E. (1975). The effects of fear appeal and communication upon attitudes toward alcohol consumption. *Journal of Drug Education, 5,* 171-181.

Giesen, M., & Hendrick, C. (1974). Effects of false positive and negative arousal feedback on persuasion. *Journal of Personality and Social Psychology, 4,* 449-457.

Gleicher, F., & Petty, R. E. (1992). Expectations of reassurance influence the nature of fear-stimulated attitude change. *Journal of Experimental Social Psychology, 28,* 86-100.

Griffin, R. J., Neuwirth, K., & Dunwoody, S. (1995). Using the theory of reasoned action to examine the health impact of risk messages. *Communication yearbook 18,* 201-228.

Grimley, D. M., Riley, G. E., Bellis, J. M., Prochaska, J. O. (1993). Assessing the stages of change and decision-making for contraceptive use for the prevention of pregnancy, sexually transmitted diseases, and acquired immunodeficiency syndrome. *Health Education Quarterly, 20,* 455-470.

Harris, M. B. (1998). *Basic statistics for behavioral science research* (2nd ed.). Boston: Allyn & Bacon.

Harris, V. A., & Jellison, J. M. (1971). Fear-arousing communications, false physiological feedback, and the acceptance of recommendations. *Journal of Experimental Social Psychology, 7,* 269-279.

Hendrick, C., Giesen, M., & Borden, R. (1975). False physiological feedback and persuasion: Effect of fear arousal vs. fear reduction on attitude change. *Journal of Personality, 43,* 196-214.

Hewgill, M. A., & Miller, G. R. (1965). Source credibility and response to fear-arousing communications. *Speech Monographs, 32,* 95-101.

Higbee, K. L. (1969). Fifteen years of fear arousal: Research on threat appeals: 1953-1968. *Psychological Bulletin, 6,* 426-444.

Horowitz, I. A. (1969). Effects of volunteering, fear arousal, and number of communications on attitude change. *Journal of Personality and Social Psychology, 11,* 34-37.

Horowitz, I. A., & Gumenik, W. E. (1970). Effects of the volunteer subject, choice, and fear arousal on attitude change. *Journal of Experimental and Social Psychology, 6,* 293-303.

Hovland, C., Janis, I., & Kelly, H. (1953). *Communication and persuasion.* New Haven, CT: Yale University.

HPV in perspective. (1991, Winter). *HPV News, 1,* 4-7.

Insko, C. A., Arkoff, A., & Insko, V. M. (1965). Effects of high and low fear-arousing communications upon opinions toward smoking. *Journal of Experimental Social Psychology, 1,* 256-266.

Janis, I. L. (1967). Effects of fear arousal on attitude change: Recent developments in theory and experimental research. In L. Berkowitz (Ed.), *Advances in experimental social psychology* (Vol. 3, pp. 166-225). New York: Academic Press.

Janis, I. L., & Feshbach, S. (1953). Effects of fear-arousing communications. *The Journal of Abnormal and Social Psychology, 48,* 78-92.

Janis, I. L., & Mann, L. (1965). Effectiveness of emotional role-playing in modifying smoking habits and attitudes. *Journal of Experimental Research in Personality, 1,* 84-90.

Janz, N., & Becker, M. (1984). The health belief model: A decade later. *Health Education Quarterly, 11,* 1-47.

Jepson, C., & Chaiken, S. (1990). Chronic issue-specific fear inhibits systematic processing of persuasive communications. *Journal of Social Behavior and Personality, 5,* 61-84.

Kelly, J. A., St. Lawrence, J. S., Diaz, Y. E., Stevenson, L. Y., Hauth, A. C., Brasfield, T. L., Kalichman, S. C., Smith, J. E., & Andrew, M. E. (1991). HIV risk behavior reduction following intervention with key opinion leaders of population: An experimental analysis. *American Journal of Public Health, 81(2),* 168-171.

Kirscht, J. P., Becker, M. H., Haefner, D. P., & Maiman, L. A. (1978). Effects of threatening communications and mothers' health beliefs on weight change in obese children. *Journal of Behavioral Medicine, 1,* 147-157.

Kirscht, J. P., & Haefner, D. P. (1973). Effects of repeated threatening health communications. *International Journal of Health Education, 16,* 268-277.

Kline, K. (1995). *Applying Witte's Extended Parallel Process Model to pamphlets urging women to engage in BSE: Where are the efficacy messages?* Paper presented at the annual meeting of the Speech Communication Association, San Antonio, TX.

Klohn, L. S., & Rogers, R. W. (1991). Dimensions of the severity of a health threat: The persuasive effects of visibility, time of onset, and rate of onset on young women's intentions to prevent osteoporosis. *Health Psychology, 10,* 323-329.

Kohn, P. M., Goodstadt, M. S., Cook, G. M., Sheppard, M., & Chan, G. (1982). Ineffectiveness of threat appeals about drinking and driving. *Accident Analysis and Prevention, 14,* 457-464.

Kok, G. (1983). The further away, the less serious: Effect of temporal distance on perceived value and probability of a future event. *Psychological Reports, 52,* 531-535.

Kotler, P. (1984). Social marketing of health behavior. In L. W. Frederikson, L. J. Solomon, & K. A. Brehony (Eds.), *Marketing health behavior* (pp. 23-39). New York: Plenum Press.

Kotler, P., & Roberto, E. (1989). Social marketing. New York: Free Press.

Knowles, J. (1994). *HPV & genital warts: Questions and answers.* NY: Planned Parenthood.

Krueger, R. A. (1988). *Focus groups: A practical guide for applied research.* Newbury Park, CA: Sage Publications.

LaTour, M. S., & Pitts, R. E. (1989). Using fear appeals in advertising for AIDS prevention in the college-age population. *Journal of Health Care Marketing, 9,* 5-14.

Lefebvre, R. C., & Flora, J. A. (1988). Social marketing and public health intervention. *Health Education Quarterly, 15,* 299-315.

Lemieux, R., Hale, J. L., & Mongeau, P. A. (1994, November). *Reducing risk behaviors related to sun exposure: The effects of fear appeals, vividness, and message framing.* Paper presented at the annual meeting of the Speech Communication Association, New Orleans.

Leventhal, H. (1970). Findings and theory in the study of fear communications. In L. Berkowitz (Ed.), *Advances in Experimental Social Psychology* (Vol. 5, pp. 119-186). New York: Academic Press.

Leventhal, H. (1971). Fear appeals and persuasion: The differentiation of a motivational construct. *American Journal of Public Health, 61,* 1208-1224.

Leventhal, H., Jones, S., & Trembly, G. (1966). Sex differences in attitude and behavior change under conditions of fear and specific instructions. *Journal of Experimental Social Psychology, 2,* 387-399.

Leventhal, H., & Niles, P. (1964). A field experiment on fear arousal with data on the validity of questionnaire measures. *Journal of Personality, 32,* 459-479.

Leventhal, H., & Niles, P. (1965). Persistence of influence for varying durations of exposure to threat stimuli. *Psychological Reports, 16,* 223-233.

Leventhal, H., & Perloe, S. I. (1962). A relationship between self-esteem and persuasibility. *Journal of Abnormal and Social Psychology, 64,* 385-388.

Leventhal, H., & Singer, R. P. (1966). Affect arousal and positioning of recommendations in persuasive communications. *Journal of Personality and Social Psychology, 4,* 137-146.

Leventhal, H., Singer, R., & Jones, S. (1965). Effects of fear and specificity of recommendation upon attitudes and behavior. *Journal of Personality and Social Psychology, 2,* 20-29.

Leventhal, H., & Trembly, G. (1968). Negative emotions and persuasion. *Journal of Personality, 36,* 154-168.

Leventhal, H., & Watts, J. (1966). Sources of resistance to fear-arousing communications on smoking and lung cancer. *Journal of Personality, 34,* 155-175.

Leventhal, H., Watts, J., & Pagano, F. (1967). Effects of fear and instructions on how to cope with danger. *Journal of Personality and Social Psychology, 3,* 313-321.

Ley, P., Bradshaw, P. W., Kincey, J. A., Couper-Smartt, J., & Wilson, M. (1974). Psychological variables in the control of obesity. In W. D. Burland, P. D. Samuel, & J. Yudkin (Eds.), *Obesity Symposium* (pp. 316-337). London: Churchhill Livingstone.

Liberman, A., & Chaiken, S. (1992). Defensive processing of personally relevant health messages. *Personality and Social Psychology Bulletin, 18,* 669-679.

Lundy, R. M., Simonson, N. R., & Landers (1967). Conformity, persuasibility, and irrelevant fear. *Journal of Communication, 27,* 39-54.

Maibach, E. W., & Cotton, D. (1995). Moving people to behavior change: A staged social cognitive approach to message design. In E. W. Maibach & R. L. Parrott (Eds.) *Designing health messages,* (pp. 41-64). Thousand Oaks, CA: Sage.

McCrosky, J. C., & Wright, D. W. (1971). A comparison of the effects of punishment-oriented and reward-oriented messages in persuasive communications. *The Journal of Communication, 21,* 83-93.

McGuire, W. J., & Parrott, R. (1995). *Designing health messages: Approaches from communication theory and public health practice.* Thousand Oaks, CA: Sage.

McGuire, W. J. (1984). Public communication as a strategy for inducing health-promoting behavioral change. *Preventive Medicine, 13,* 299-319.

McGuire, W. J. (1985). Attitudes and attitude change. In L. Gardner and E. Aronson (Eds.), *Handbook of Social Psychology: Volume 2* (3rd ed.), (pp. 233-346). New York: Random House.

Mewborn, C. R., & Rogers, R. W. (1979). Effects of threatening and reassuring components of fear appeals on physiological and verbal measures of emotion and attitudes. *Journal of Experimental Social Psychology, 15,* 242-253.

Meyer, G. (1997). *An introduction to evaluating HIV prevention programs.* Michigan Department of Community Health. Lansing, MI.

Meyer, G., & Dearing, J. W. (1996, Winter). Respecifying the social marketing model for unique populations. *Social Marketing Quarterly.*

Meyerowitz, B. E., & Chaiken, S. (1987). The effect of message framing on breast self-examination attitudes, intentions, and behavior. *Journal of Personality and Social Psychology, 52,* 500-510.

Nisbett, R. E., & Ross, L. (1980). *Human inference: Strategies and shortcomings of social judgment.* Englewood Cliffs, NJ: Prentice Hall.

Norman, N. M., & Tedeschi, J. T. (1989). Self-presentation, reasoned action, and adolescents' decisions to smoke cigarettes. *Journal of Applied Social Psychology, 19,* 543-558.

Perkins, K. A., & Scott, R.R. (1986). A low-cost environmental intervention for reducing smoking among cardiac inpatients. *The International Journal of the Addictions, 21,* 1173-1182.

Petty, R. E., & Cacioppo, J. T. (1986). The elaboration likelihood model of persuasion. In L. Berkowitz (Ed.), *Advances in Experimental Social Psychology* (Vol. 19, pp. 123-205).

Powell, F. A. (1965). The effect of anxiety-arousing messages when related to personal, familial, and impersonal referents. *Speech Monographs, 32,* 102-106.

Powell, F. A., & Miller, G.R. (1967). Social approval and disapproval cues in anxiety-arousing communications. *Speech Monographs, 34,* 152-159.

Prentice-Dunn, S., & Rogers, R. W. (1986). Protection motivation theory and preventive health: Beyond the health belief model. *Health Education Research, 1,* 153-161.

Prochaska, J. O., DiClemente, C. C., & Norcross, J. C. (1992). In search of how people change: Applications to addictive behaviors. *American Psychologist, 47,* 1102-1114.

Prohaska, T. R., Keller, M. L., Leventhal, E. A., & Leventhal, H. (1987). The impact of symptoms and aging attributions on emotions and coping. *Health Psychology, 6,* 495-514.

Ramirez, A., & Lasater, T. L. (1977). Ethnicity of communicator, self-esteem, and reactions to fear-arousing communications. *The Journal of Social Psychology, 102,* 79-91.

Reeves, B. R., Newhagen, J., Maibach, E., Basil, M., & Kurz, K. (1991). Negative and positive television messages: Effects of message type and context on attention and memory. *American Behavioral Scientist, 34,* 679-694.

Rhodes, P., & Wolitski, R. J. (1990). Perceived effectiveness of fear appeals in AIDS education: Relationship to ethnicity, gender, age, and group membership. *AIDS Education and Prevention, 2,* 1-11.

Rice, R., & Atkin, C. K. (1989). *Public communication campaigns,* (2nd ed.). Newbury Park, CA: Sage.

Rice, R., & Atkin, C. K. (2001). *Public communication campaigns* (3rd ed.). Thousand Oaks, CA: Sage.

Rippetoe, P. A., & Rogers, R. W. (1987). Effects of components of protection-motivation theory on adaptive and maladaptive coping with a health threat. *Journal of Personality and Social Psychology, 52,* 596-604.

Robberson, M. R., & Rogers, R. W. (1988). Beyond fear appeals: Negative and positive persuasive appeals to health and self-esteem. *Journal of Applied Social Psychology, 18,* 277-287.

Roberto, A. J., Meyer, G., Atkin, C. K., & Johnson, A. J. (2000). Using the Extended Parallel Process Model to prevent firearm injury and death: Field experiment results of a video-based intervention. *Journal of Communication.*

Roberto, A. J., Meyer, G., Boster, F. J., & Story, H. L. (2000). Adolescents' decisions about verbal and physical aggression: An application of the Theory of Reasoned Action. Manuscript submitted for publication.

Rodriguez, J. I. (1995). *Confounds in fear arousing persuasive messages: Do the paths less traveled make all the difference?* Unpublished doctoral dissertation, Michigan State.

Rogers, E. M. (1995). *Diffusion of Innovations.* (4th ed.). New York: The Free Press.

Rogers, E. M., & Bhowmik, D. K. (1971). Homophily-heterophily: Relational concepts for communication research. *Public Opinion Quarterly, 34,* 523-538.

Rogers, R. W. (1975). A protection motivation theory of fear appeals and attitude change. *Journal of Psychology, 91,* 93-114.

Rogers, R. W. (1983). Cognitive and physiological processes in fear appeals and attitude change: A revised theory of protection motivation. In J. Cacioppo & R. Petty (Eds.), *Social Psychophysiology* (pp. 153-176). New York: Guilford.

Rogers, R. W., & Deckner, C.W. (1975). Effects of fear appeals and physiological arousal upon emotion, attitudes, and cigarette smoking. *Journal of Personality and Social Psychology, 32,* 222-230.

Rogers, R. W., & Mewborn, C. R. (1976). Fear appeals and attitude change: Effects of a threat's noxiousness, probability of occurrence, and the efficacy of the coping responses. *Journal of Personality and Social Psychology, 34,* 54-61.

Rook, K. (1986). Encouraging preventive behavior for distant and proximal health threats: Effects of vivid versus abstract information. *Journal of Gerontology, 41,* 526-534.

Rosen, T. J., Terry, N. S., & Leventhal, H. (1982). The role of esteem and coping in response to a threat communication. *Journal of Research in Personality, 16,* 90-107.

Rosenstock, I. M. (1974). The health belief model and preventive health behavior. *Health Education Monographs, 2,* 354-386.

Schwarz, N., Servay, W., & Kumpf, M. (1985). Attribution of arousal as a mediator of the effectiveness of fear-arousing communications. *Journal of Applied Social Psychology, 15,* 178-188.

Self, C. A., & Rogers, R. W. (1990). Coping with threats to health: Effects of persuasive appeals on depressed, normal, and antisocial personalities. *Journal of Behavioral Medicine, 13,* 343-357.

Shelton, M. L., & Rogers, R. W. (1981). Fear-arousing and empathy-arousing appeals to help: The pathos of persuasion. *Journal of Applied Social Psychology, 11,* 366-378.

Simonson, N. R., & Lundy, R. M. (1966). The effectiveness of persuasive communication presented under conditions of irrelevant fear. *Journal of Communication, 16,* 32-37.

Skilbeck, C., Tulips, J., & Ley, J. (1977). The effects of fear arousal, fear position, fear exposure, and sidedness on compliance with dietary instructions. *European Journal of Social Psychology, 7,* 221-239.

Smart, R. G., & Fejer, D. (1974). The effects of high and low fear messages about drugs. *Journal of Drug Education, 4,* 225-235.

Smith, M. J. (1977). The effects of threat to attitudinal freedom as a function of message quality and initial receiver attitude. *Communication Monographs, 44,* 196-206.

Smith, S. W., Kopfman, J. M., Morrison, K., & Ford, L. A. (1993, May). *The effects of message sidedness, fear, and prior thought and intent on the memorability and persuasiveness of organ donor card message strategies.* Paper presented at the annual meeting of the International Communication Association, Washington, DC.

Stainback, R., & Rogers, R. W. (1983). Identifying effective components of alcohol abuse prevention programs: Effects of fear appeals, message style, and source expertise. *The International Journal of the Addictions, 18,* 393-405.

Stephenson, M. T. (1993). *A subliminal manipulation of the extended parallel process model.* Unpublished master's thesis, Texas A&M University.

Stewart, C. J., & Cash, W. B., Jr. (2000). *Interviewing: Principles and practices.* New York: McGraw Hill.

Stout, P. A., & Sego, T. (1994b, July). *The role of need for cognition in response to threat appeals in AIDS messages.* Paper presented at the annual meeting of the Speech Communication Association.

Struckman-Johnson, C. J., Gilliland, R. C., Struckman-Johnson, D. L., & North, T. C. (1990). The effects of fear of AIDS and gender on responses to fear-arousing condom advertisements. *Journal of Applied Social Psychology, 20,* 1396-1410.

Sutton, S. R., & Eiser, J. R. (1984). The effects of fear-arousing communications on cigarette smoking: An expectancy-value approach. *Journal of Behavioral Medicine, 7,* 13-33.

Sutton, S. R, & Hallett, R. (1989a). The contribution of fear and cognitive factors in mediating the effects of fear-arousing communications. *Social Behaviour, 4,* 83-98.

Sutton, S. R., & Hallett, R. (1989b). Understanding seat-belt intentions and behavior: A decision-making approach. *Journal of Applied Social Psychology, 19,* 1310-1325.

Tanner, J. F., Day, E., & Crask, M. R. (1989). Protection motivation theory: An extension of fear appeals theory in communication. *Journal of Business Research, 19,* 267-276.

Vanlandingham, M. J., Suprasert, S., Grandjean, N., Sittitrai, W. (1995). Two views of risky sexual practices among northern Thai males: The health belief model and the theory of reasoned action. *Journal of Health and Social Behavior, 36,* 195-212.

Webster's New World College Dictionary (4th ed.) (1999). New York: McMillan.

Weinstein, N. D. (1980). Unrealistic optimism about future life events. *Journal of Personality and Social Psychology, 39,* 806-820.

Weinstein, N. D. (1982). Unrealistic optimism about susceptibility to health problems. *Journal of Behavioural Medicine, 5,* 441-460.

Weinstein, N. D. (1988). Precaution adoption process. *Health Psychology, 7,* 355-386.

Williams, R. E., Ward, D. A., & Gray, L. N. (1985). The persistence of experimentally induced cognitive change: A neglected dimension in the assessment of drug prevention programs. *Journal of Drug Education, 15,* 33-42.

Witte, K. (1991). *Preventing AIDS through persuasive communications: Fear appeals and preventive-action efficacy.* Unpublished doctoral dissertation, University of California, Irvine.

Witte, K. (1992a). Putting the fear back into fear appeals: The extended parallel process model. *Communication Monographs, 59,* 329-349.

Witte, K. (1992b). The role of threat and efficacy in AIDS prevention. *The International Quarterly of Community Health Education, 12,* 225-249.

Witte, K. (1992c). Preventing AIDS through persuasive communications: A framework for constructing effective, culturally-specific, preventive health messages. *International and Intercultural Communication Annual, 16,* 67-86.

Witte, K. (1994). Fear control and danger control: A test of the Extended Parallel Process Model (EPPM). *Communication Monographs, 61,* 113-134.

Witte, K. (1995). Fishing for success: Using the persuasive health message framework to generate effective campaign messages. In E. Maibach & R. Parrott (Eds.), *Designing health messages: Approaches from communication theory and public health practice* (pp. 145-166). Thousand Oaks, CA: Sage.

Witte, K. (1997). Preventing teen pregnancy through persuasive communications: Realities, myths, and the hard-fact truths. *Journal of Community Health, 22*(2), 137-154.

Witte, K. (1998). Fear as motivator, fear as inhibitor: Using the EPPM to explain fear appeal successes and failures. In P. A. Andersen and L. K. Guerrero (Eds.), *The Handbook of Communication and Emotion* (pp. 423-450). New York: Academic Press.

Witte, K., & Allen, M. (in press). A meta-analysis of fear appeals: Implications for effective public health campaigns. *Health Education & Behavior.*

Witte, K., Berkowitz, J., Lillie, J., Cameron, K., Lapinski, M. K., & Liu, W. Y. (1998). Radon awareness and reduction campaigns for African-Americans: A theoretically-based formative and summative evaluation. *Health Education and Behavior, 25,* 284-303.

Witte, K., Cameron, K. A., McKeon, J., & Berkowitz, J. (1996). Predicting Risk Behaviors: Development and Validation of a Diagnostic Scale. *Journal of Health Communication, 1,* 317-341.

Witte, K., & Morrison, K. (2000). Examining the influence of trait anxiety/repression-sensitization on individuals' reactions to fear appeals. *Western Journal of Communication, 64,* 1-29.

Witte, K., Murray, L., Hubbell, A. P., Liu, W. Y., Sampson, J., Morrison, K. (in press). Addressing cultural orientation in fear appeals: Promoting AIDS-protective behaviors among Hispanic immigrants and African-American adolescents, and American and Taiwanese college students. *Journal of Health Communication.*

Witte, K., Nzyuko, S., & Cameron, K. (1995). *HIV/AIDS along the Trans-Africa Highway in Kenya: Examining risk perceptions, recommended responses, and campaign materials.* Preliminary report for the AURIG, Michigan State University.

Witte, K., Stokols, D., Ituarte, P., & Schneider, M. (1993). A test of the perceived threat and cues to action constructs in the health belief model: A field study to promote bicycle safety helmets. *Communication Research, 20,* 564-586.

Yin, R. K. (1988). Case study research: Design and methods. Newbury Park, CA: Sage.

Suggested Readings

Beach, R. I. (1966, June). The effect of a "fear-arousing" safety film on physiological, attitudinal, and behavioral measures: A pilot study. *Research Review,* pp. 53-57.

Beck, K. H. (1984). The effects of risk probability, outcome severity, efficacy of protection and access to protection on decision making: A further test of Protection Motivation Theory. *Social Behavior and Personality, 12,* 121-125.

Ben-Sira, Z. (1981). Latent fear-arousing potential of fear-moderating and fear-neutral health promoting information. *Social Science and Medicine, 15e,* 105-112.

Boer, H., & Seydel, E. (1996). Protection motivation theory. In M. Connor and P. Norman (Eds.), *Predicting health behavior: Research and practice with social cognition models* (pp. 95-120). Buckingham, PA: Open University Press.

Boyle, G. J. (1984). Effects of viewing a road trauma film on emotional and motivational factors. *Accident Analysis and Prevention, 16,* 383-386.

Brown, R. A. (1979). Fear-induced attitude change as a function of conformity and drinking pattern in alcoholics. *Journal of Clinical Psychology, 35,* 454-456.

Calantone, R. J., & Warshaw, P. R. (1985). Negating the effects of fear appeals in election campaigns. *Journal of Applied Psychology, 70,* 627-633.

Carey, J. C. (1990). *The influence of involvement on cognitive and emotional responses to fear appeals.* Unpublished master's thesis, University of Texas, Austin.

Chang, J. L. (1989). *Emotional response and the use of threat appeals.* Unpublished master's thesis, University of Texas, Austin.

Covello, V., von Winterfeldt, D., & Slovic, P. (1986). Risk communication: A review of the literature. *Risk Abstracts, 3,* 171-182.

DeWolfe & Governale. (1964). Fear and attitude change. *Journal of Abnormal and Social Psychology, 69,* 119-123.

Dillard, J. P., Plotnick, C. A., Godbold, L. C., Freimuth, V. S., & Edgar, T. (1996). The multiple affective outcomes of AIDS PSAs: Fear appeals do more than scare people. *Communication Research, 23,* 44-72.

Dziokonski, W., & Weber, S. J. (1977). Repression-sensitization, perceived vulnerability, and the fear appeal communication. *The Journal of Social Psychology, 102,* 105-112.

Evans, R. I., Rozelle, R. M., Lasater, T. M., Dembroski, T. M., & Allen, B. P. (1970). Fear arousal, persuasion, and actual versus implied behavioral change: New perspective utilizing a real-life dental hygiene program. *Journal of Personality and Social Psychology, 2,* 220-227.

Finckenauer, J. O. (1982). *Scared straight and the panacea phenomenon.* Englewood Cliffs, NJ: Prentice Hall.

Fruin, D. J., Pratt, C., & Owen, N. (1992). Protection motivation and adolescents' perceptions of exercise. *Journal of Abnormal Social Psychology, 22,* 55-69.

Geller, E. S. (1989). Using television to promote safety belt use. In R. E. Rice and C. K. Atkin (Eds.), *Public communication campaigns* (pp. 201-203). Newbury Park, CA: Sage.

Goldstein, M. J. (1959). The relationship between coping and avoiding behavior and response to fear-arousing propaganda. *Journal of Abnormal and Social Psychology, 58,* 247-252.

Griffeth, R. W., & Rogers, R. W. (1976). Effects of fear-arousing components of driver education on students' safety attitudes and simulator performance. *Journal of Educational Psychology, 68,* 501-506.

Haefner, D. P. (1956). Some effects of guilt-arousing and fear-arousing persuasive communications on opinion change. *Abstracts American Psychologist, 11,* 359.

Haefner, D. P. (1965). Arousing fear in dental health education. *Journal of Public Health Dentistry, 25,* 140-146.

Hale, J., & Mongeau, P. (1991, May). *Testing a causal model of the persuasive impact of fear appeals.* Paper presented at the annual meeting of the International Communication Association, Chicago.

Hale, J. L., & Dillard, J. P. (1995). Fear appeals in health campaigns: Too much, too little, or just right? In E. Maibach, and R. L. Parrott (Eds.), *Designing health messages* (pp. 65-80). Thousand Oaks, CA: Sage.

Hale, J. L., Lemieux, R., & Mongeau, P. A. (1995). Cognitive processing of fear-arousing message content. *Communication Research, 22,* 459-474.

Hale, J. L., Mongeau, P. A., & Lemieux, R. (1993, November). *Trait anxiety and fear-arousing messages regarding sun exposure.* Paper presented at the annual meeting of the Speech Communication Association, Miami Beach, FL.

Hass, J. W., Bagley, G. S., & Rogers, R. W. (1975). Coping with the energy crisis: Effects of fear appeals upon attitudes toward energy consumption. *Journal of Applied Psychology, 60,* 754-756.

Hill, D., & Gardner, G. (1980). Repression-sensitization and yielding to threatening health communications. *Australian Journal of Psychology, 32,* 183-193.

Horowitz, I. A. (1972). Attitude change as a function of perceived arousal. *The Journal of Social Psychology, 87,* 117-126.

Hunter, J. E., & Schmidt, F. L. (1990). *Methods of meta-analysis.* Newbury Park, CA: Sage.

Janis, I. L., & Feshbach, S. (1954). Personality differences associated with responsiveness to fear-arousing communications. *Journal of Personality, 23,* 154-166.

Janis, I. L., & Terwilliger, R. F. (1962). An experimental study of psychological resistance to fear arousing communications. *Journal of Abnormal and Social Psychology, 65,* 403-410.

Job, R.F.S. (1988). Effective and ineffective use of fear in health promotion campaigns. *American Journal of Public Health, 78,* 163-167.

Kantola, S. J., Syme, G. J., & Nesdale, A. R. (1983). The effects of appraised severity and efficacy in promoting water conservation: An informational analysis. *Journal of Applied Social Psychology, 13,* 164-182.

Kazoleas, D., & Linmon, M. (1997). *Designing effective fear based health campaigns: Testing the ability of qualitative evidence to derail counterargument generation.* Paper presented at the Central States Communication Association Convention, St. Louis, MO.

Kendall, C., & Hailey, B. (1993). The relative effectiveness of three reminder letters on making and keeping mammogram appointments. *Behavioral Medicine, 19,* 29-34.

Keesling, B. J., & Friedman, H. (1991). *Interventions to prevent skin cancer: Experimental evaluation of informational and fear appeals.* Unpublished manuscript.

Kim, M., & Hunter, J. (1993a). Attitude-behavior relations: A meta-analysis of attitudinal relevance and topic, *Journal of Communication, 43,* 101-143.

Kim, M., & Hunter, J. (1993b). Relationships among attitudes, behavioral intentions, and behavior: A meta-analysis of past research, Part II. *Communication Research, 20,* 331-364.

Kleinot, M. C., & Rogers, R. W. (1982). Identifying effective components of alcohol misuse prevention programs. *Journal of Studies on Alcohol, 43,* 802-811.

Krisher, H. P., III, Darley, S. A., & Darley, J. M. (1973). Fear-provoking recommendations, intentions to take preventive actions, and actual preventive actions. *Journal of Personality and Social Psychology, 26,* 301-308.

Larson, E. B., Bergman, J., Heidrich, F., et al. (1982). Do postcard reminders improve influenza vaccination compliance? *Med Care, 20,* 639-648.

LaTour, M. S., Snipes, R., & Bliss, S. (1996, March/April). Don't be afraid to use fear appeals: An experimental study. *Journal of Advertising Research, 28,* 59-67.

Maddux, J. E., & Rogers, R. W. (1983). Protection motivation and self-efficacy: A revised theory of fear appeals and attitude change. *Journal of Experimental Social Psychology, 19,* 469-479.

McGuire, W. J. (1968). Personality and susceptibility to social influence. In E. Borgatta and W. Lambert (Eds.), *Handbook of personality theory and research* (pp. 1130-1187). Chicago: Rand McNally.

McGuire, W. J. (1969). The nature of attitudes and attitude change. In G. Lindzey & E. Aronson (Eds.), *The handbook of social psychology* (Vol. 3, pp. 136-314). Reading, MA: Addison-Wesley.

Miller, G. R. (1963). Studies on the use of fear appeals: A summary and analysis. *Central States Speech Journal, 14,* 117-125.

Moltz, H., & Thislethwaite, D. L. (1955). Attitude modification and anxiety reduction. *Journal of Abnormal and Social Psychology, 50,* 231-237.

Mongeau, P. (1994). Another look at fear arousing persuasive appeals. In M. Allen & R. Preiss (Eds.), *Prospects and precautions in the use of meta-analysis* (pp. 75-100). Dubuque, IA: William C. Brown.

Mulilis, J-P., Lippa, R. (1990). Behavioral change in earthquake preparedness due to negative threat appeals: A test of protection motivation theory. *Journal of Applied Social Psychology, 20,* 619-638.

O'Keefe, D. J. (1990). *Persuasion: Theory and research.* Newbury Park, CA: Sage.

Piggot, T. (1994). Methods for handling missing data in research synthesis. In H. Cooper and L. Hedges (Eds.), *The handbook of research synthesis* (pp. 163-175). New York: Russell Sage Foundation.

Radelfinger, S. (1965). Some effects of fear-arousing communications on preventive health behavior. *Health Education Monographs, 19,* 2-15.

Ragsdale, J., & Durham, K. (1986). Audience response to religious fear appeals. *Review of Religious Research, 28,* 40-50.

Ramirez, A., & Laster, T. L. (1976). Attitudinal and behavioral reactions to fear-arousing communications. *Psychological Reports, 38,* 811-818.

Ray, M. L., & Wilkie, W. L. (1970). Fear: The potential of an appeal neglected by marketing. *Journal of Marketing, 34,* 54-62.

Rogers, R. W. (1985). Attitude change and information integration in fear appeals. *Psychological Reports, 56,* 179-182.

Rogers, R. W., Deckner, C. W., & Mewborn, C. R. (1978). An expectancy-value theory approach to the long-term modification of smoking behavior. *Journal of Clinical Psychology, 34,* 562-566.

Rogers, R. W., & Thislethwaite, D. L. (1970). Effects of fear arousal and reassurance on attitude change. *Journal of Personality and Social Psychology, 15,* 227-233.

Schwarzer, R., & Fuchs, R. (1996). Self-efficacy and health behaviors. In M. Connor and P. Norman (Eds.), *Predicting health behavior: Research and practice with social cognition models* (pp. 165-195). Buckingham: Open University Press.

Shepard, B., Hartwick, J., & Warshaw, P. (1988). A theory of reasoned action: A meta-analysis of past research with recommendations for modifications and future research. *Journal of Consumer Research, 5,* 325-343.

Sherer, M., & Rogers, R. W. (1984). The role of vivid information in fear appeals and attitude change. *Journal of Research in Personality, 18,* 321-334.

Siero, S., Kok, G., & Pruyn, J. (1984). Effects of public education about breast cancer and breast self-examination. *Social Science and Medicine, 18,* 881-888.

Smalec, J. (1996). *Bulimia interventions via interpersonal influence: The role of threat and efficacy in persuading bulimics to seek help.* Paper presented at the Speech Communication Association Convention, San Diego, CA.

Smith, S. L. (1996, May). *The effective use of fear appeals in persuasive immunization messages: An analysis of national immunization intervention messages.* Paper presented at the annual meeting of the International Communication Association, Chicago.

Stanley, M. A., & Maddux, J. E. (1986). Cognitive processes in health enhancement: Investigation of a combined protection motivation and self-efficacy model. *Basic and Applied Social Psychology, 7,* 101-113.

Stephenson, M. T., & Witte, K. (1997). *Fear, threat, and perceptions of efficacy from frightening skin cancer messages.* Paper presented at the annual meeting of the International Communication Association, Montreal.

Sternthal, B., & Craig, C. S. (1974). Fear appeals: Revisited and revised. *Journal of Consumer Research, 1,* 22-34.

Stout, P. A., & Sego, T. (1994a). Emotions elicited by threat appeals and their impact on persuasion. In K. King (Ed.), *Proceedings of the 1994 Conference of the American Academy of Advertising* (pp. 8-16). Athens GA: American Academy of Advertising.

Stout, P. A., & Sego, T. (1995). Response to threat appeals in public service announcements. In C. Madden (Ed.), *Proceedings of the 1995 Conference of the American Academy of Advertising* (pp. 78-86). Athens, GA: American Academy of Advertising.

Sturges, J., & Rogers, R. (1996). Preventive health psychology from a developmental perspective: An extension of protection motivation theory. *Health Psychology, 15,* 158-166.

Sutton, S. R. (1982). Fear-arousing communications: A critical examination of theory and research. In J. R. Eiser, J.R. (Ed.), *Social psychology and behavioral medicine* (pp. 303-337). London: Wiley.

Sutton, S. R., & Hallett, R. (1988). Understanding the effects of fear-arousing communications: The role of cognitive factors and amount of fear aroused. *Journal of Behavioral Medicine, 11,* 353-360.

Van der Velde, F. W., & Van der Pligt, J. (1991). AIDS-related behavior: Coping, protection motivation, and previous behavior. *Journal of Behavioral Medicine, 14,* 429-451.

Walsh, D. C., Hingson, R. W., Merrigan, D. M., Levenson, S. M., Coffman, G. A., Heeren, T., & Cupples, A. (1992). The impact of a physician's warning on recovery after alcoholism treatment. *Journal of the American Medical Association, 267,* 663-667.

Watson, M., Pettingale, K. W., & Goldstein, D. (1983). Effects of fear appeal on arousal, self-reported anxiety, and attitude towards smoking. *Psychological Reports, 52,* 139-146.

Weinstein, N. D., Sandman, P. M., & Roberts, N.E. (1990). Determinants of self-protective behavior: Home radon testing. *Journal of Applied Social Psychology, 20,* 783-801.

Wheatley, J. J., & Oshikawa, S. (1970). The relationship between anxiety and positive and negative advertising appeals. *Journal of Marketing Research, 7,* 85-89.

Witte, K. (1993). Message and conceptual confounds in fear appeals: The role of threat, fear, and efficacy. *Southern Communication Journal, 58,* 147-155.

Witte, K., Berkowitz, J., Cameron, K., & Lillie, J. (1998). Preventing the spread of genital warts: Using fear appeals to promote self-protective behaviors. *Health Education & Behavior, 25,* 571-585.

Witte, K., & Morrison, K. (1995). The use of scare tactics in AIDS prevention: The case of juvenile detention and high school youth. *Journal of Applied Communication Research, 23,* 128-142.

Witte, K., Peterson, T. R., Vallabhan, S., Stephenson, M. T., Plugge, C. D., Givens, V. K., Todd, J. D., Becktold, M. G., Hyde, M. K., & Jarrett, R. (1993). Preventing tractor-related injuries and deaths in rural populations: Using a Persuasive Health Message (PHM) framework in formative evaluation research. *International Quarterly of Community Health Education, 13,* 219-251.

Wolf, S., Gregory, W. L., & Stephan, W. G. (1986). Protection motivation theory: Prediction of intentions to engage in anti-nuclear war behaviors. *Journal of Applied Social Psychology, 16,* 310-321.

Wunsch, J. M. (1996). Perceived threat of cancer and perceived efficacy of fruit and vegetable intake in reducing cancer risk by participants in a WIC program. Manuscript under review.

Wurtele, S. (1988). Increasing women's calcium intake: The role of health beliefs, intentions, and health value. *Journal of Applied Social Psychology, 18,* 627-639.

Wurtele, S., & Maddux, J.E. (1987). Relative contributions of protection motivation theory components in predicting exercise intentions and behavior. *Health Psychology, 6,* 453-466.

Index

About the Authors

KIM WITTE (PhD, University of California) is professor in the Department of Communication at Michigan State University. Her current research focuses on the development of effective health risk messages for members of diverse cultures. Dr. Witte is the chair of the Health Communication Division of the International Communication Division and a past chair of the Health Communication Division of the National Communication Association. She sits on 10 editorial boards and has served as expert consultant to the National Libraries of Medicine, the Centers for Disease Control and Prevention (CDC), the National Institute of Occupational Safety and Health (NIOSH), and other agencies. Her work has appeared in *Social Science and Medicine, International Quarterly of Communication Health Education, Communication Yearbook, Health Education & Behavior, Communication Monographs*, and *Journal of Community Health*, among other publications. Dr. Witte has received funding from the CDC, NIOSH, the American Cancer Society, and others. Her work has been recognized by more than a dozen "Top Paper" awards at both national and international conferences, as well as by the "Distinguished Article Award" from the Applied Communication Division of the National Communication Association, in recognition of the applied and practical value of her research. In 1997, Dr. Witte was awarded the "Teacher-Scholar Award" from Michigan State University, in recognition of excellence in research and undergraduate education. Recently, Dr. Witte was named the *Lewis Donohew Outstanding Scholar in Health Communication*, in recognition of her outstanding research contributions to the health communication field during the preceding biennium.

GARY MEYER (PhD, Michigan State University) is assistant professor in the Department of Communication Studies at Marquette University in Milwaukee, Wisconsin. His primary research focuses on health communication in the areas of health promotion and disease prevention. Dr. Meyer has been an investigator for the Agency for Health Care Policy and Research as well as the U.S. Environmental Protection Agency, and has been published in the *Journal of Health Communication, Journal of Communication, Communication Research, Science Communication*, and *Social Marketing Quarterly*. He has received a Telly Award (1998) for his work in the area of violence prevention and has been named Outstanding New Teacher (1999) by the Central States Communication Association.

DENNIS MARTELL (PhD) is a health educator and Director of the Center for Sexual Health Promotion at Michigan State University, where he supervises the HIV/AIDS Counseling and Testing Center. He has a B.S. in biology, M.A. in health education, M.A. in family therapy, and Ph.D. in family dynamics and human sexuality. Dr. Martell also teaches human sexuality in the Department of Psychology at Lansing Community College. He is a well-respected educator and researcher in the area of health promotion and has been involved nationally in numerous conferences, presentations, television productions, and publications.

Printed in the United Kingdom
by Lightning Source UK Ltd.
129841UK00001BA/3-8/A